European Oncology Leaders

The CancerFutures Collection
2001–2004

European Oncology Leaders

The CancerFutures Collection 2001–2004

With 140 Figures

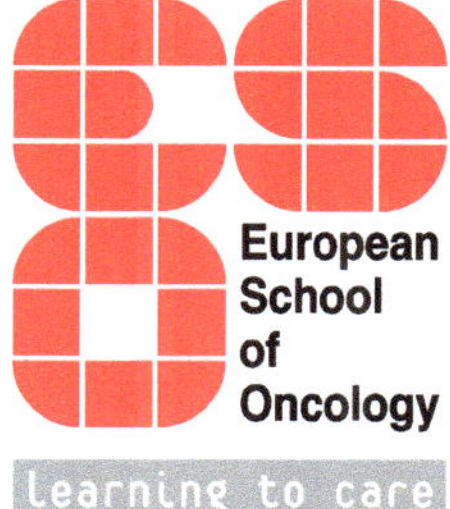

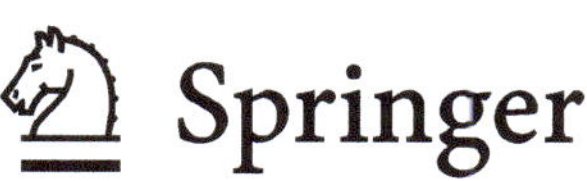

Springer

Professor Umberto Veronesi
Dr. Kathy Redmond

European School of Oncology

Viale Beatrice d'Este, 37
20122 Milan, Italy
eso@esoncology.org
www.cancerworld.org

ISBN 3-540-23658-9

Springer-Verlag
Berlin Heidelberg NewYork

Library of Congress Control Number:
2004113915

The use of general descriptive names, registered names, trademarks, etc. in this publication does not imply, even in the absence of a specific statement, that such names are exempt from the relevant protective laws and regulations and therefore free for general use.

Product liability: The publishers cannot guarantee the accuracy of any information about dosage and application contained in this book. In every individual case the user must check such information by consulting the relevant literature.

Editor: Dr. Rolf Lange, Heidelberg
Desk Editor: Hiltrud Wilbertz, Heidelberg
Typsetting: SDS, Leimen
Production: Bernd Reichenthaler,
Pro Edit GmbH, Heidelberg
Printing: ABC-Druck, Heidelberg
Binding: Schäffer, Grünstadt

Springer is a part
of Springer Science+Business Media
springeronline.com

Printed on acid-free paper
27/3150/Re – 543210

Contents

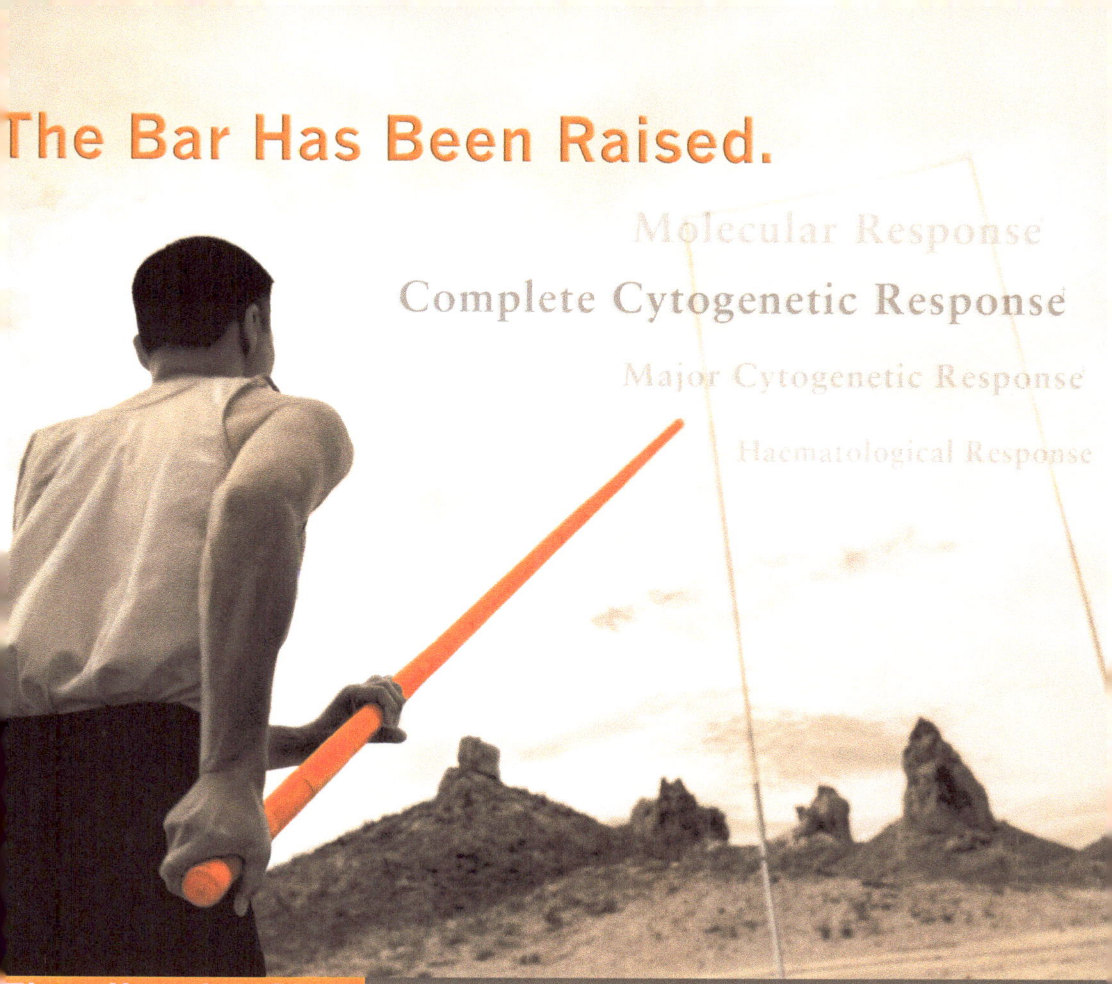

The Bar Has Been Raised.

First-line for CML

Glivec® is indicated for the treatment of patients with newly diagnosed Philadelphia chromosome (*bcr-abl*) positive (Ph+) chronic myeloid leukaemia (CML) for whom bone marrow transplantation is not considered as the first line of treatment.

www.glivec.com

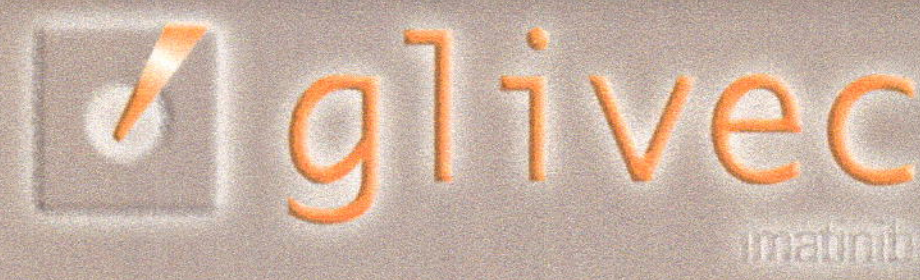

After 12 months of Glivec therapy, 39% of patients with a complete cytogenetic response (elimination of the Philadelphia chromosome) had achieved a molecular response (>3 log reduction in *bcr-abl*), detected by quantitative RT-PCR.[1]

After 18 months of Glivec therapy, 76% of patients were estimated by Kaplan-Meier analysis to have achieved a complete cytogenetic response.[2]

After 18 months of Glivec therapy, 87% of patients were estimated by Kaplan-Meier analysis to have achieved a major cytogenetic response ($\leq$35% Ph+ cells).[2]

Please see Summary of Product Characteristics at www.glivec.com

References: 1. Hughes T, Kaeda J, Branford S, et al. Molecular responses to imatinib (STI571) or interferon + Ara-C as initial therapy for CML: results in the IRIS study. Blood. 2002;100:93a. Abstract 345. 2. O'Brien SG, Guilhot F, Larson RA, et al. Imatinib compared with interferon and low-dose cytarabine for newly diagnosed chronic-phase chronic myeloid leukemia. N Engl J Med. 2003;348:994-1004.

GLIVEC® Hard capsules

Presentation: Imatinib mesilate. Capsules containing 100 mg of imatinib as mesilate. **Indications:** Treatment of patients with newly diagnosed chronic myeloid leukaemia (CML) as well as for the treatment of patients with CML in blast crisis, accelerated phase, or in chronic phase after failure of interferon-alpha therapy. Treatment of adult patients with unresectable and/or metastatic, malignant gastrointestinal stromal tumours (GIST). **Dosage:** Adults: 400 mg a day for patients in chronic phase CML and 600 mg a day for patients in accelerated phase or blast crisis, administered orally once daily. Children: 260 mg/m² daily for chronic phase CML and 340 mg/m² daily for advanced phase CML. The total daily dose in children not to exceed adult equivalent doses of 400 and 600 mg. Adults: 400 mg a day for patients with unresectable and/or metastatic, malignant GIST. Potential need for dose adjustment due to side-effects or insufficient response to therapy. **Contraindications:** Hypersensitivity to imatinib or to any of the excipients. **Precautions/Warnings:** Should be taken with food and a large glass of water to minimise the risk of gastrointestinal disturbances. Caution in patients with hepatic or severe renal impairment, or a history of cardiac disease. Beware of severe fluid retention. It is recommended that patients be weighed regularly. Regular monitoring of complete blood counts and liver function tests. No experience in children below the age of three. Should not be used during pregnancy unless clearly necessary. Should not be used by breast-feeding mothers. **Interactions:** Caution with concomitant use of drugs inhibiting or inducing CYP3A4 (eg, ketoconazole, dexamethasone, rifampicin, simvastatin), or being substrates of CYP3A4 (eg, cyclosporin, paracetamol) or CYP2D6. **Adverse reactions:** Most common undesirable effects are: headache, nausea, vomiting, diarrhoea, dyspepsia, abdominal pain, myalgia, muscle spasm and cramps, dermatitis, eczema, rash, oedema, fluid retention, fatigue, neutropenia, thrombocytopenia, anaemia. **Packs and prices:** Country-specific. **Note:** Before prescribing, consult full product information.

Introduction

U. VERONESI and K. REDMOND

CancerFutures was launched in 2001 with the aim of increasing knowledge about the complex world of cancer care through people and facts. Cover Story and Masterpiece are two key sections of the magazine that have featured in-depth interviews with some of Europe's most influential oncology leaders-people who have been pioneers of the art and science of oncology over the past 30 years. These interviews comprise a unique collection of stories that give insight into the many personal and professional challenges these leaders have faced in building their careers and pushing forward the boundaries of oncology practice.

The European School of Oncology has been a proud supporter of CancerFutures since its establishment and is pleased to launch the CancerFutures Collection – a compilation of interviews that will be of interest to all members of the European oncology community, both today and in the future. This collection has allowed us to acknowledge the tremendous contribution that these leaders have made to cancer care and pay tribute to their dedication and drive. The CancerFutures Collection provides a permanent testament to their work and vision. It will provide encouragement for all those confronted with difficulties in building their careers, and perhaps, will

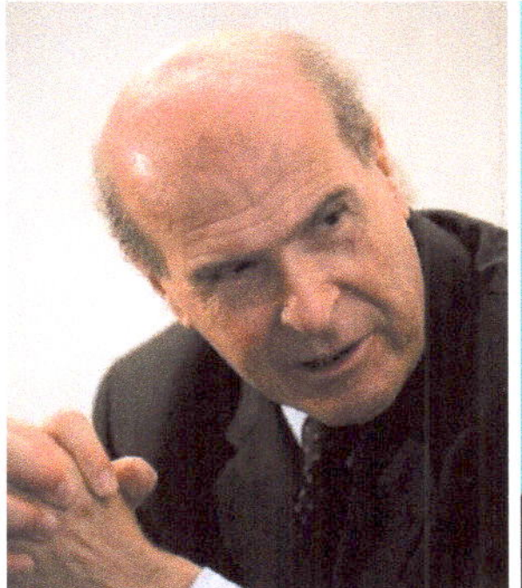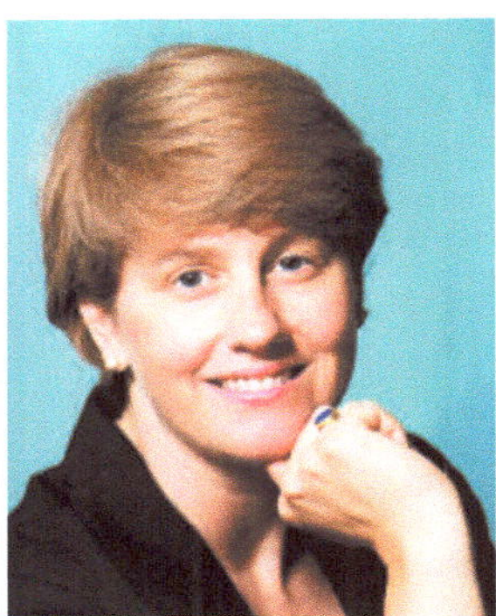

Umberto Veronesi, Chairman of the Scientific Committee, European School of Oncology, Milan (left); Kathy Redmond, Editor CancerWorld, Milan (right)

give some inspiration for our future leaders.

We would like to thank all those who have contributed to this work – the oncology leaders for agreeing to be interviewed, the journalists who carried out the interviews and the many people who were involved in the production process. We also would like to thank some of the people behind CancerFutures – particularly, Professor Maurice Schneider, Editor-in-Chief, for his leadership and Alberto Costa, who had the idea, not only for the magazine, but also for the Cover Story section. We hope that readers will enjoy this special collection of cancer stories and gain new knowledge from the myriad experience and insights of an exceptional group of people.

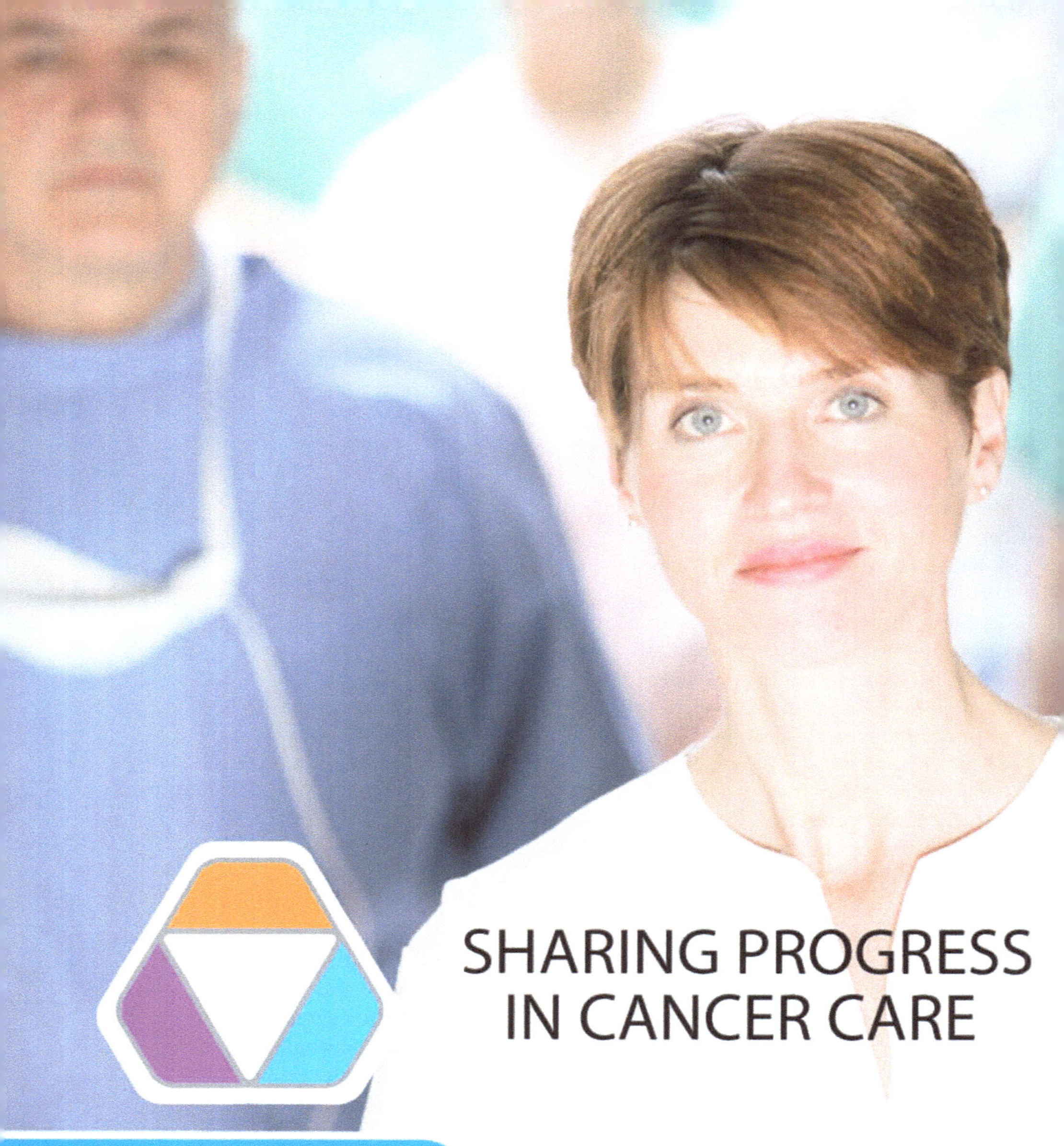

SHARING PROGRESS IN CANCER CARE

The magazine CancerWorld and the Masterclass in Clinical Oncology are two pioneer initiatives of the European School of Oncology (ESO) financially supported through Sharing Progress in Cancer Care. This is a collaborative programme between ESO and some of the world's leading pharmaceutical companies including Amgen, AstraZeneca, Aventis, Eli Lilly, Merck, Novartis and Roche.

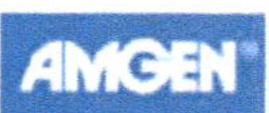

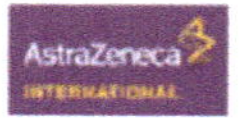

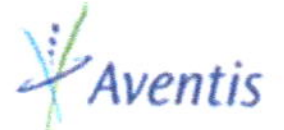

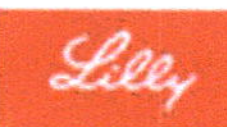

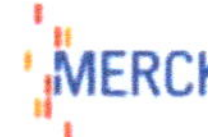

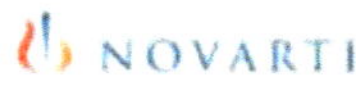

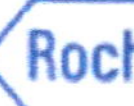

Cover Stories

Martine Piccart: Medic and Musician...

Helen Saul

At the opening ceremony of the second European Breast Cancer Conference, Brussels, September 2000, Professor Martine Piccart gave, as expected, a highly polished scientific speech. Then she walked across to the piano and performed a couple of movements from a Smetana trio, accompanied by her daughters. Two played, on cello and violin, while the youngest turned the pages at the piano. The audience was first taken aback and later spellbound. Afterwards, and after the applause, Piccart returned to the podium and coolly mediated a discussion. One delegate muttered, "Now she'll probably go home and cook a six course meal for them all..."

Martine Piccart is a consummate all-rounder. She is a top European oncologist, head of chemotherapy at the Jules Bordet Institute in Brussels and associate professor in oncology. She is also a pianist, trained to professional level, and she has apparently managed to nurture similar talent in her daughters.

She specialises in breast and ovarian cancer and is a member of numerous international oncology and cancer research organisations, a teacher at European and American institutions and a frequent speaker at international symposia. At the moment she is engaged in the small matter of changing the nature of clinical trials in Europe; but more of that later.

Piccart made key decisions early on. Her father was a gynaecologist and saw patients at home, so she was always aware of his work. By the time she was eight years old, she had decided to study medicine herself. She started playing the piano at around the same time and she flourished both in her academic work and her music. By her late teens, she was in a position to choose between a career as a pianist and, as best student of her year at school, in medicine. She chose the latter and has not regretted it.

A family tragedy sowed the seeds of her decision to study oncology. When she was 12 years old, her great-uncle was treated for colon cancer at the Jules Bordet Institute, where she

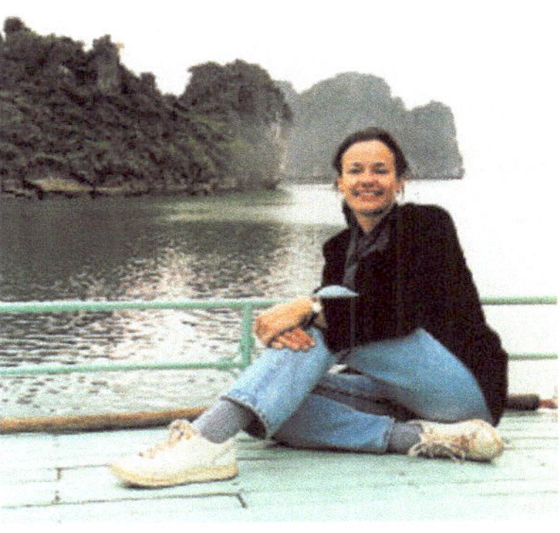

Martine Piccart
in Vietnam

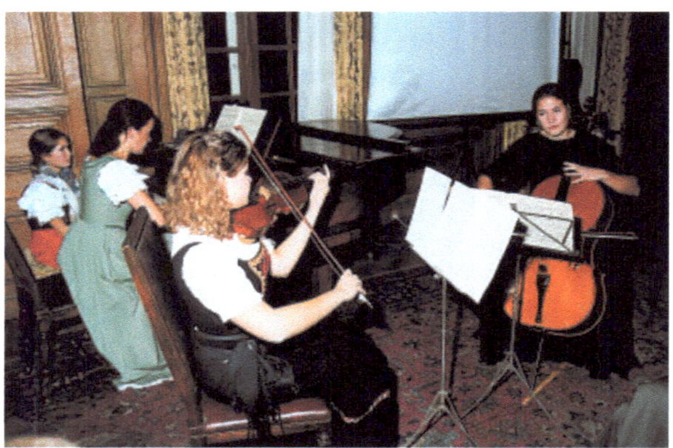

now works. "When I came to visit my uncle, at that moment, something happened. Something about the hospital impressed me and when I started medicine I already had it in my mind to do oncology", she says. Sadly, her uncle died, but apart from a brief flirtation with the idea of paediatrics, she stuck with her initial choice. Later career decisions were also influenced by personal experience, though she says not consciously. A friend's mother died of ovarian cancer shortly before she embarked on her fellowship in New York; her own mother survived breast cancer 20 years ago. She herself is at high risk of the disease, "and of course I have three daughters". Even the naturally-driven need incentives; this is clearly powerful.

"I am certainly not a discoverer, I am not going to find a new drug or molecular pathway. My contribution is more in putting people

Piccart studied medicine at the Free University of Brussels where she met Michael Gebhart, from Germany, a fellow medical student and violinist. He was looking for someone to practice with, was introduced to Piccart and together they staged

concerts to raise money for cancer research. She laughs now at their idealism at the time, yet she still displays much of the optimism more characteristic of students (her most over-used words in this interview were "lucky" and "fantastic"). And of course, she is still playing to benefit cancer research.

In the end, she graduated not only with "La plus grande distinction" and the Fleuris Mercier Award for the best medical student, but also having met her future husband. She and Gebhart, an orthopaedic surgeon, have now been married for 21 years. They still play tennis together twice a week and, incidentally, their eldest daughter Geraldine has just completed her first year at medical school.

So Piccart worked in Brussels, took a two-year fellowship in New York, then returned to the Jules Bordet Institute, where she has been ever since, steadily building both her own and her department's reputation. It seems so neat, so ordered - have there been no setbacks?

She admits that arriving in New York "was quite a difficult time". This, it turns out, is something of an understatement. Both she and Gebhart had to find a fellowship in the same place, which was not easy, and the timing was even worse: their second daughter, Laurence, was only nine days old when they arrived the States. Piccart's original placement turned out to be an hour and a half's journey from where they were living, with on-call duties in the evenings and weekends. Gebhart's work involved long hours and, with two very young children, it was impossible.

However, with hallmark determination, she managed to rearrange

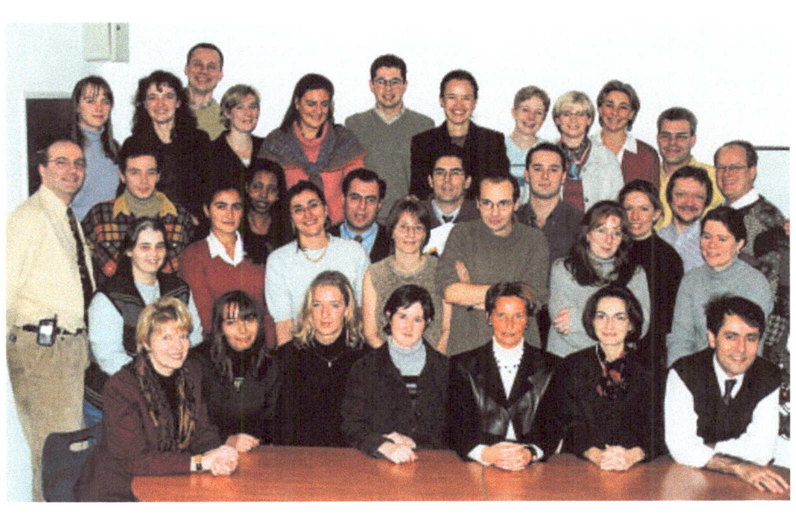

her fellowship and worked for two years with Professor Franco Muggia at the New York University Medical Center. This involved fewer clinical duties, more time for real research and opportunities for travel. She "opened her mind completely" to new ideas and got to know American oncologists personally, which has facilitated collaboration ever since. It was pivotal to her career, she says, "a real enrichment" and she tries to offer young fellows in her department the same opportunities. In fact, her number one piece of advice to young oncologists is to leave their institution and spend two or three years abroad.

Once back in Brussels, she worked for Professor J. Klastersky, head of internal medicine at Jules Bordet, who gave her the freedom to develop her priorities. She sees patients two days a week and spends the rest - the other four days, she says - in research. Her department has grown from 10 to 30 and her own standing has risen. She won the European Society of Medical Oncology Award in 1997 for her "ex-

ceptional contribution ... to the advancement of medical oncology in Europe, in particular in the fields of breast cancer and ovarian cancer". She was thrilled.

But out of this star-studded background, how exactly has she advanced medical oncology? What has she brought to the field that is unique?

Communication and collaboration is at the heart of her work, and she says, "I am certainly not a discoverer, I am not the person who is going to find a new drug against cancer or a fantastic new molecular pathway. My contribution is more into trying to put people together and stimulate them to work together." In this she is the latest in a long and eminent line at Jules Bordet. Her mentor in the early years, Marcel Rozencweig, was himself a pupil of Henri Tagnon, founder of the European Organization for Research and Treatment of Cancer (EORTC), originally based at Jules Bordet. Emanuel Vanderschueren, a later EORTC president, also impressed her. She says she "grew up with the EORTC" and with the idea that international cooperation and collaboration is the way ahead. She chaired the EORTC treatment division for three years and is still a member of its gynaecological cancer study group, breast cancer cooperative group and early clinical studies group.

> **"Large adjuvant studies carried out by pharmaceutical companies can be extremely powerful and good, but data should still preferably be analysed by independent bodies."**

Now, though, much of her energy is devoted to BIG, the Breast International Group, and Piccart's baby, and it is through BIG that she hopes to change our approach to clinical trials in cancer. It started five years ago when she was invited by American Society of Clinical Oncology (ASCO) to discuss the role of adjuva therapy for breast cancer in postmenopausal women. This meant reviewing all the trials that had been done. "I was really disappointed. I thought the type of research we currently do in Europe in early breast cancer is not at all satisfactory. There are many many trials with a similar design, all too small and underpowered. I thought we must be able to do much better if we get together."

At the same time, she was becoming concerned that the pharmaceutical industry is increasingly carrying out the good, large trials. "I felt a danger there for the future of cancer research. I thought that if they are going to start doing the large adjuvant studies, it is probably not in the best interests of science and patients. They can be extremely powerful and

good, the trials they run are now of very high standards. But the data should preferably still be analysed by independent bodies."

The answer, she thought, lies first in formal collaboration between research groups throughout Europe, and then in close links with the pharmaceutical industry. She received immediate and strong support from the internationally renowned breast cancer expert, Professor Aron Goldhirsch, head of medical oncology at the European Cancer Institute in Milan. She then nervously invited the heads of 20 European research groups round a table. Most were immediately enthusiastic about the idea, and BIG was born.

Now, at BIG meetings, a research group can present an idea for a trial. It is discussed, suggestions made and sometimes the design improved. All other groups are invited to join, but there is no obligation, and the trial is run by a designated coordinating group. At present, seven studies are up and running, another four set to start and many more under discussion.

> **"We cannot afford to spend eight years testing one drug and then move on.
> We need to find a better way, and I am hoping BIG is it."**

BIG trials are often run in partnership with pharmaceutical companies, which can involve a meeting of two quite distinct cultures. But both have something to offer. The companies frequently own the drugs to be tested, while BIG represents large numbers of patients and the chance of faster accrual into trials. Piccart believes that the key to the success of the partnership is that data are collected and analysed by the independent researchers in the BIG group. Companies collaborate closely and have access to the efficacy data in full once trials are completed.

This model of collaboration comes at a crunch time for clinical research, she says. "We are going to have, in the coming years, many interesting molecules that have to be tested in subsets of patients. That means screening many times more patients before entry into the trial, because only a proportion will have tumours expressing the target protein. We need to do these trials rapidly, we can not afford to spend eight years on one drug and then move on. We need to find a better way, and I am hoping BIG is it."

The BIG model is starting to spread. Similar groups have been set up for other cancers, notably ovarian and colorectal cancer. Other disciplines could also benefit: BIG aims to use research grants from pharmaceutical companies to support trials in radiotherapy and surgery, which are a lot more difficult to fund.

> **"Laboratory scientists have discovered fantastic things about how cancer cells survive and resist treatment, while oncologists have kept doing boring studies comparing treatments A and B"**

So what next? Well, there's the business of "inducing a complete change in mentality" among oncologists. "It's a real pity. Over the last 15 or 20 years we have not been talking to laboratory scientists enough. We have gone our way while they were

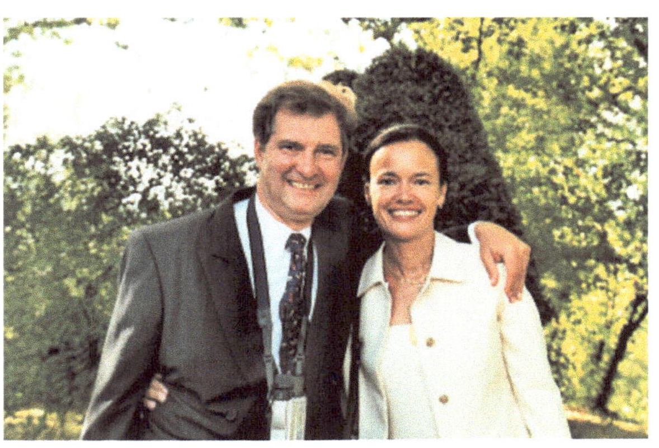

Martine Piccart with husband Michael Gebhart

discovering fantastic things regarding the way a cancer cell survives and resists chemotherapy and hormonal therapy and so on. We have kept doing relatively boring studies comparing treatment A versus treatment B but we have not tried to understand why treatment A works in 60% of the population and treatment B in perhaps 40%. So the next challenge is going to be to reinforce this dialogue with fundamental research and to start clinical studies to test hypotheses generated by lab research."

Oncologists are becoming more receptive to this, because new microarray technology, which provides a picture of the genes expressed in an individual tumour, is likely to help explain why some tumours respond well to drug A and some others don't. But she says it is not going to be easy to put into practice. "The problem is that you need to get a biopsy of the tumour under very specific conditions, which takes time. You need to motivate your surgeon, your pathologist, and your institute, so it's a different way of functioning. It is really difficult to get busy oncologists enthusiastic about this and to accept the extra effort, but this is what we

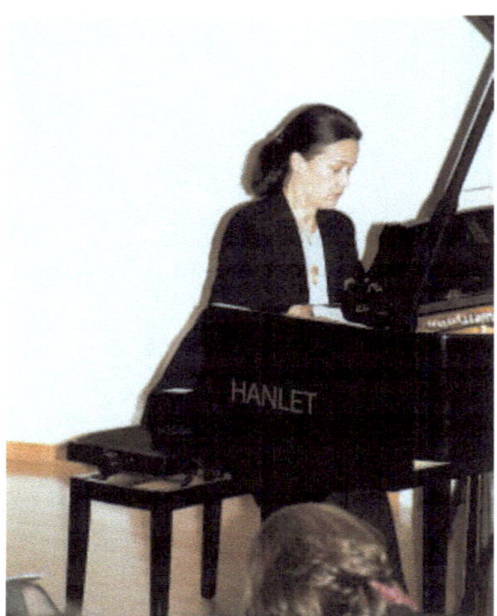

At the piano

will have to do in future. It will be absolutely essential to continuing progress in oncology, and 10 to 15 years from now we will no longer see trials of the kind we see today. At least that is what I am hoping."

"Ten to 15 years from now we will no longer see trials of the kind we see today. At least that is what I am hoping."

Along these lines, one BIG-EORTC study is testing the laboratory-generated hypothesis that the taxanes are only useful to patients whose tumour has a mutated p53 protein. It will involve 1,300 patients, compared to more than 24,000 already contributing to trials of taxanes in early breast cancer which have so far provided no clear answer. Piccart: "If this relatively small trial verifies the hypothesis, we will probably witness a kind of revolution in clinical trials. This trial will or will not work, but for sure in the very near future we will have better tools and will be able to correlate patterns of gene expression with the efficacy or lack of it, of treatments.

I want BIG to push this type of research a lot more."

Piccart is not the only oncologist to be calling for more collaboration between groups, or for a greater emphasis on translational research. Even BIG is not an original idea, in that it is based on a model she saw working in the States. But she is one of the few who are taking these ideas and making them happen in Europe. Bringing different research groups together, or persuading different disciplines to cooperate takes a certain rather specific talent, and a colleague says she is simply "exceptionally gifted". The monthly teleconference meetings can be quite tense, as opinions compete and sometimes collide. "She has an incredible ability to focus on the issue and draw out the main points. She holds things together while always being diplomatic. It's very rare."

"She has an incredible ability to focus on the issue and draw out the main points. She holds things together while always being diplomatic. It's very rare."

Piccart herself says often that she has been lucky. Lucky in the people who trained her, lucky in the institute which encouraged her to do clinical research from her first year in oncology, lucky in her experience in the States, lucky now in her boss and her team. And maybe she has been. But she has also been determined, brave and unswerving in her goals. In the nicest possible – collaborative – way.

Piccart occasionally plays in a quartet with her two eldest daughters and her husband, who has switched now from violin to viola. Somehow it comes as little surprise when she says that Brahms is one of her favourite composers of chamber music. Because, she says, "There is a dialogue going on between instruments which is very nice. Sometimes, with other composers, the piano or another instrument can dominate. But in Brahms' music they each have their role." A bit like cancer researchers, really.

Gordon McVie: Making Waves

HELEN SAUL

Professor Gordon McVie keeps a painting in his office, given to him by a former patient. The painting is of sailing ships and she said it reminded her of him. When asked in what way, she replied that as he came striding through the ward, his white coat always flew out behind him like sails in the wind. He likes to move at speed.
Many years after dropping the ward rounds, first for academia, and later to become Director General of the UK's Cancer Research Campaign (CRC), the image lingers. Tall and confident, an imposing figure, McVie is still in a hurry. Though he's perhaps not so much harnessing the wind these days as making waves himself.

McVie has become the unofficial chief advocate for UK cancer patients, and it is a role which fits him well. He is a master of the media soundbite and has a rare talent for being able to describe the most technical of research advances in 15 seconds dead. Genetics, microbiology, functional imaging: nothing is so abstract or complicated that it cannot be packaged for a general audience. New treatments for neuroblastoma may not sound an ideal subject for daytime television, but McVie can turn it into one.

His gift for handling the media does not make him friends everywhere. McVie is not afraid of controversy and does not pull his punches, even, or maybe especially, when millions are listening. He is outspoken on subjects like research funding, tobacco advertising and patients' access to new drugs. The UK government, for one, is sensitive to any criticism on its performance on health,

and who knows what prompted it to both appoint a national cancer director to oversee the delivery of cancer services, and to state its aim of reducing cancer deaths by a fifth by 2010?

His optimism on the likely benefits of research is legendary and

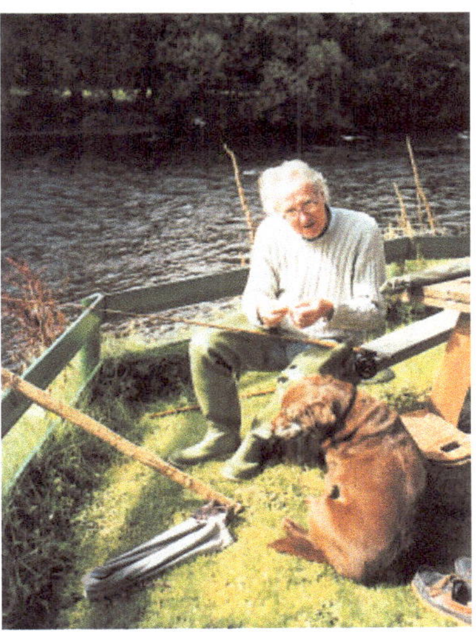

McVie: UK's chief advocate for cancer patients

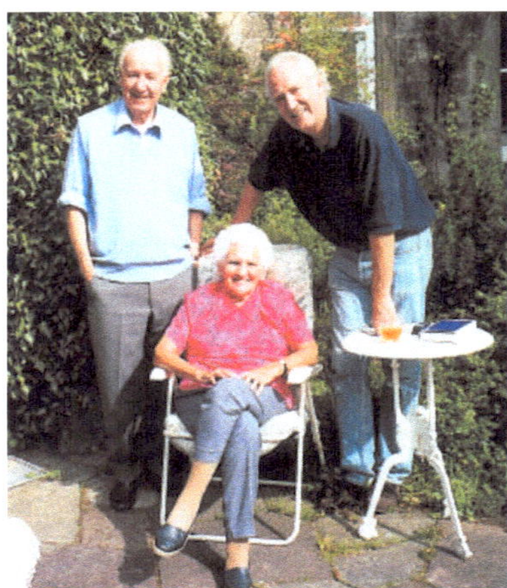

even upsets his friends. It worries scientists, perplexes clinicians and was directly attacked by the Lancet, which devoted an entire editorial to "Overoptimism about cancer". This was prompted by McVie's claims that the end to cancer is in sight, and that it will be beaten in the lifetime of his sons. It will be as readily controlled as diabetes is today, he said, and become a chronic rather than a fatal disease. Provided, of course, that sufficient resources are devoted to research. To the Lancet, such claims are "premature", "flagrant exaggeration" and may shatter the confidence of donators "when the public starts to see the gap between what is being said and what is being achieved."

> **Such claims are premature, flagrant exaggeration and may deter donators when they start to see the gap between what is being said and what is being achieved – the Lancet**

McVie shrugs. "The Lancet has every right to its own prognostication on the time it will take to de-feat cancer. I also have a right to my view." He cites his impressive track record in clinical and academic medicine and research, his position as European editor of the US Journal of the National Cancer Institute and, at CRC, the privilege of being surrounded by top scientists and clinicians. "It's my job to take a helicopter view of things from time to time, and try to work out for the sake of those people giving money to charity, what the prospects are that their money will do any good. I wasn't in the slightest bit dismayed about the Lancet's view and I'm perfectly happy to debate it."

Robust in the face of criticism, he almost seems glad that his views are getting another airing, even if to be pulled apart. But if he is not upset by the Lancet, surely he understands the concern of colleagues at the coal face? "Scientists are nervous that there might be any over-emphasis on the promise emerging from their work. I am well aware that they don't want me over-selling their stuff. But the news about cancer over the last 15 to 20 years has been generally bad: cancers are going to carry on going up, everything kills you, exhaust fumes kill you, your diet kills you, strawberries will give you this cancer, raspberries some other kind.

"If you look hard, as I do, at the outcome of the last 20 years of research, you can't come to any conclusion other than an optimistic one. We have got really solid data which say that the outcome for cancer patients in this country has improved, and that is not due to improvements in the health service. It has been due to the delivery of the products, the harvest, the fruits of cancer research."

It's a typically bullish response. McVie is not easily deflected by niggles or niceties within the scientific community, and is determined to do all he can to sell the cause of research to the public. "We have only got something like three percent of our cancer patient population in clincial trials, and that is a national disgrace. If I can do anything to persuade people that they would get better cancer treatment if they were in a clinical trial, then I am doing them a service. All the data pooled together – and there are 50 references – show quite categorically that if you are treated in a clinical trial you do better than if not, and it doesn't matter which arm of the clinical trial you are in. So until we are up to say 20 percent of the cancer population going into clinical trials, then I am not going to shut up."

McVie clearly takes seriously his responsibility to promote cancer research and to trumpet the achievements of scientists and clinicians who work on CRC subsidy. But in fact, speaking out is only part of the job at CRC. He manages the 1000 employees and 1500 scientists who receive grants indirectly through universities, and he spends much of his time whirling round the country, visiting laboratories, clinics, groups of supporters and fund-raising shops.

His job also means dealing with animal rights protests. He and his family have all received direct threats; scientists and supporters have been attacked. A parcel bomb was sent to an 83-year-old woman for no other reason than that she had supported and raised money for CRC for 40 years. "I find that absolutely despicable, totally indefensible, and if I can put myself in line, in between a supporter like that and the animal rights brigade, I will do that."

Nevertheless, his is in essence a desk job. McVie is frustrated with bureaucracy and paperwork, and is not an administrator by nature – he can lose six mobile phones in three years – but he says the high point of his time at CRC was winning an Investors in People award. "It was outstanding, the first time any major charity has won this status for an entire business. It meant that volunteers, supporters, members of staff were all valued as individuals and encouraged to grow within their jobs. It gave me a tremendous thrill."

A long way from clinical practice

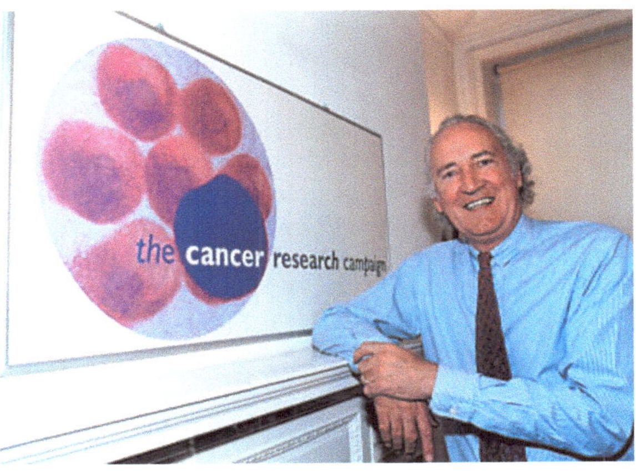

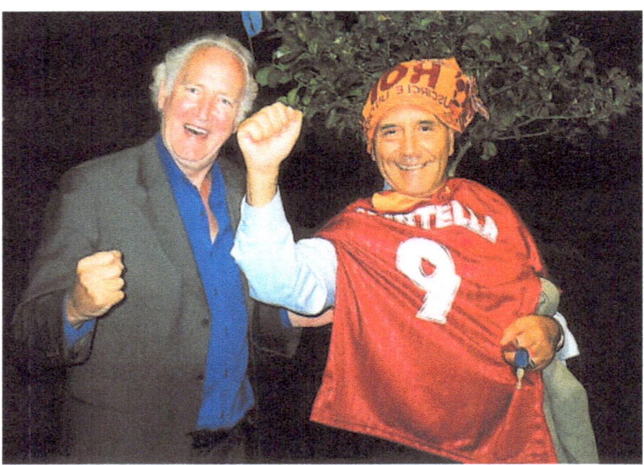

Gordon McVie and Pier Giorgio Natali, Scientific Director of the Regina Elena Cancer Institute, Rome, after Roma won the Italian League

Yet it is all a long way from the clinical practice he spent 30 years training for. He accepts rather begrudgingly that he has found his niche as a spokesman for cancer, and says, "I think I can do more good for more patients doing what I am doing now than seeing patients on a one-to-one basis for three-quarters of an hour a session." But he misses clinical medicine "big time", and says, "You know I am happy to go back to that if they decide to dump me here."

> "I can do more good for more patients doing what I am doing now than seeing patients on a one-to-one basis for three-quarters of an hour a session."

That would be unlikely under normal circumstances, but these are strange times at CRC. A merger with the UK's other major cancer charity, Imperial Cancer Research Fund (ICRF), is to proceed early in 2002. McVie and his opposite number at ICRF, Sir Paul Nurse, have been discussing the possibility for five years, and driving it through. It has now been formally announced and is re-puted to be the biggest merger in the voluntary sector, anywhere in the world, ever.

The main rationale for it, according to McVie, is to push the science on. The technology needed for research is no longer the bottleneck to progress; it is the money to pay for that technology. Both ICRF and CRC want the same technology; they are also competing for too few scientists and clinical researchers. The merger means that resources are pooled, top people shared and the administration run more efficiently. Already 186 redundant posts have been identified, which translates into considerable cost savings and makes the pound in the collecting box go that bit further.

It makes sense logically, but many have built careers at one or other of the charities, and there is healthy competition between the two. Polls suggest that supporters are overwhelmingly in favour, but many scientists, publicists and fundraisers within the organisations are feeling apprehensive. None other than McVie's wife, Claudia, who works at CRC as head of a region's fundraising, has been bitterly opposed to the merger. McVie, as one of the main architects, obviously believes in it and is not one to be deflected by criticism, even from such a close quarter. Indeed, he seems completely unruffled by it. Though he says, with a smile, that Claudia is coming round to the idea.

McVie will take charge of communications in the new charity, Cancer Research UK, while Sir Paul takes responsibility for science. The overall Chief Executive Officer will be Professor Andrew Miller, drafted in from the outside. For McVie then,

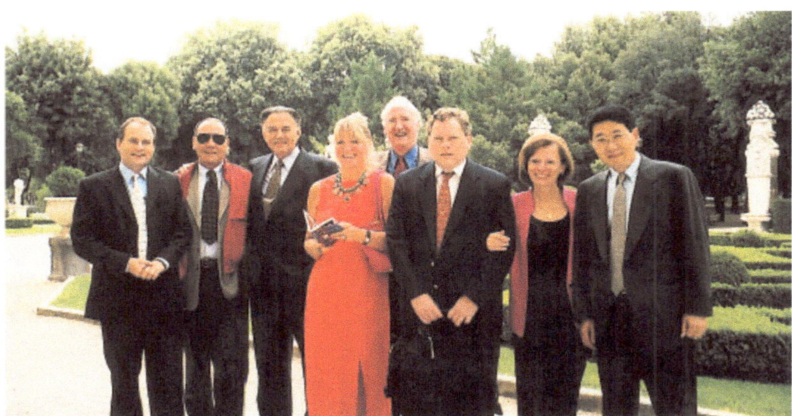

Gordon McVie (middle, back) and Claudia McVie (red dress) with other delegates to the World Alliance of Cancer Research Organizations meeting in Rome

it is one further step away from science and the clinic and one more towards his role as arguably the most high-profile spokesperson for medicine in the UK.

His route here got off to a rather shaky start. He went to a school in Edinburgh, where he was consistently less successful than his father had been. Having underperformed in comparison in every area, including classwork, sports and the cadet force, he knew only that he did not want to follow his father into law. A careers master suggested that those with marks like his, around 50 percent in most subjects, make good general practitioners, and off he went to study medicine at Edinburgh University. He was also prompted by a distressing family experience. His Auntie Jean had ovarian cancer while he was in his late teens and was nursed at home by his mother for six months. Jean, a childless widow who looked after McVie "as a spoilt brat of a nephew", opted to go into a phase I trial of mustine. "You can't think of anything more nasty to put in somebody's pleura, but she was very brave and decided to take part in this experiment. Once she

The merger with ICRF means that resources are pooled, top people shared and the administration run more efficiently. It will make the pound in the collecting box go that bit further.

got over the vomiting with mustine, it did actually improve her quality of life and I think this was an influence on me."

However, pre-clinical medicine was not to his liking. He found it sociable, but boring, a drudge. His unremarkable academic performance continued and he failed two out of three subjects in his first year. A talking-to from his parents persuaded him to stick it out, but he continued to skid along the bottom in his studies. He surprised himself – and his teachers – with excellence in a physiology exam, but was thought too unreliable to take on an honours degree. However, a pathology professor later took a risk on him and, for McVie, this was the watershed. He found out where the library was, discovered what the BMJ and Lancet looked like, and set to, writing a 3000 word essay every week on some aspect of inflammation or autoimmunity. He undertook a project in a department with a staff-to-student ratio of 6:1. "That was really terrific. I suddenly started enjoying it, suddenly thought that this is all right, I could do this. And suddenly, I became an academic. I published a paper at the end of that year in the British Journal of Clinical Pathology, and it has to be one of my most cited papers. There were 750 requests for abstracts and reprints, it was amazing," he says.

From there, he became the young doctor to watch, and a list of his mentors reads like a miniature Who's Who in British medicine. Sir Derek Dunlop (later of the Dunlop Committee on Therapeutics in Medicine) and his successor, Ronald Girdwood, persuaded him, as a houseman, to apply for a Government Medical Research Council (MRC) Research Fellowship. His application, for research into the immunology of Hodgkin's disease, was successful and he went on to spend seven years as a lecturer in Sir Derek's department. McVie so impressed Professor Gordon Hamilton Fairley at St Bartholomew's Hospital, London, then the only medical oncologist in the UK, that Hamilton Fairley arranged for him to visit the United States and work at different

McVie was President of EORTC from 1994 to 1997

departments over several months. Hamilton Fairley was killed by an IRA bomb, an event which McVie says could have ended his career flat, but which instead inspired him to achieve. In any case, Hamilton Fairley's influence persisted after his death; he had advised CRC to set up chairs in medical oncology in Manchester, Cambridge, Glasgow and Southampton. The Glasgow chair went to surgeon Sir Kenneth Calman (later chief medical officer of Scotland, then of England and Wales — he gives his name to the Calman-Hine model for cancer centres in the UK, and also to junior hospital training). He needed a senior lecturer with experience in medical oncology, and McVie was the only person in Scotland who was trained. At 31, he got the job, and became the first consultant in medical oncology in the whole of Scotland.

For the next five years, with 12 beds, he and Calman were responsible for all cancer patients in a population of 2.5 million in the West of Scotland. It was an enormous commitment and left little time for research. He wrote a number of project grant applications and pulled in scientists to help with research, but could not carry it out himself.

Eventually, he decided that in order to think about his next step, to concentrate on new drugs, pharmacology and pharmacokinetics, he would have to go somewhere where English was not spoken. It was the only way to prevent himself being tempted back into clinical rounds. He took a three-month sabbatical at the Netherlands Cancer Institute, Amsterdam, and stayed there nine years. He again had a 12-bed unit, but this time it was only for phase

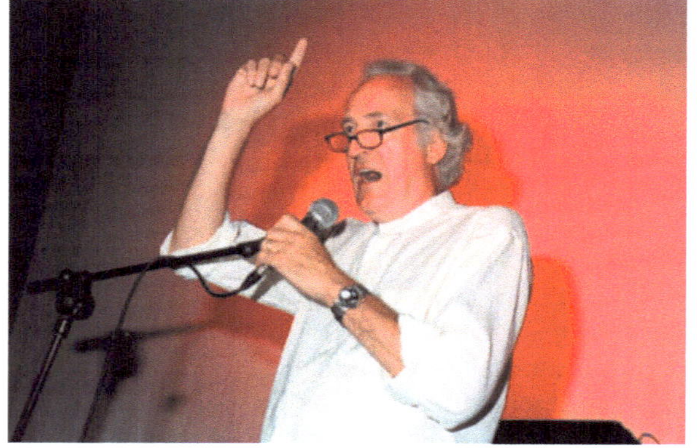

I clinical trials, and he was given a laboratory to continue working in clinical pharmacology and drug discovery. These were productive years, and he became Clinical Research Director at the Institute. He remained there until he was offered the position of Scientific Director at CRC, back in London, and in April 1996, of Director General.

From 1994 to 1997, he was also President of EORTC (European Organisation for Research and Treatment of Cancer), which he says taught him the beginnings of diplomacy. "I learned how to balance the views and the expectations of people from different countries in Europe, and I became much more skilled than I ever was before in handling discussions between disciplines."

If CRC has nurtured his campaigning side, it has also moved his personal life on. His first marriage started to crumble while he was in Amsterdam, and he met Claudia through CRC. They were married three years ago, walking away from the ceremony to James Brown's "I Feel Good". They are enjoying life together and have no problem relaxing away from work, whether it's through opera, theatre, wine or food. McVie's three rugby-playing sons, two of whom are junior Scottish nationals ("that talent seems to have skipped a generation"), live in Scotland, but Claudia's two children from her first marriage live nearer and visit often. The McVies have a dog and a cat and have both just bought golf clubs and taken up the sport. "We'll see how that goes…", he says.

But what for the future? His career seems to be moving inexorably into the public domain and away

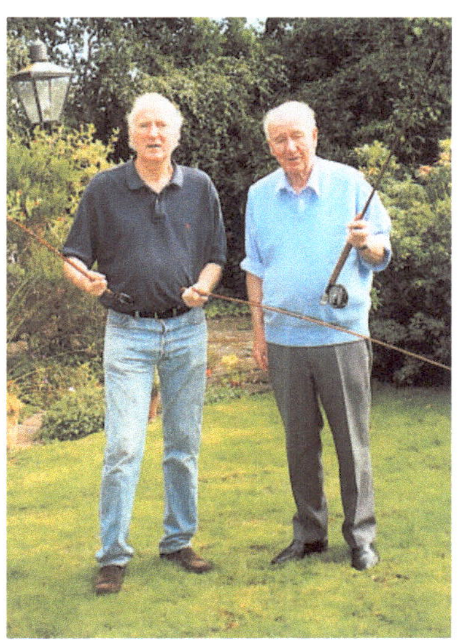

Showing off fishing gear with McVie senior

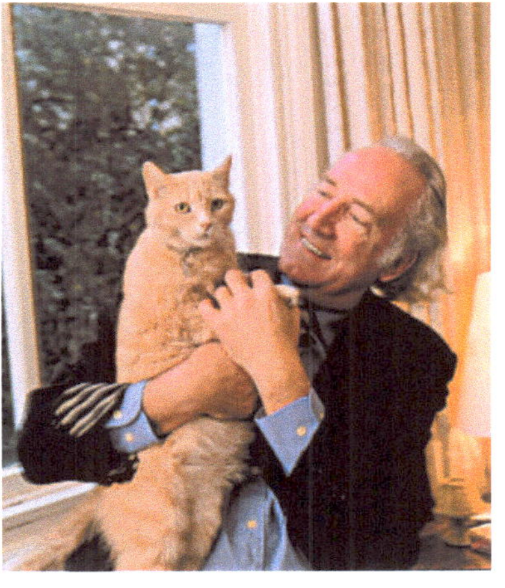

McVie has always kept both cats and dogs

from the clinic, and the division of responsibilities at the new charity, Cancer Research UK, will exaggerate this further. As befits the product of a high Tory father and a socialist mother, he has no political affiliation. He is a defender of the right to free care at the point of access, and of free education. But his interest in politics is pragmatic, in trying to make systems work. He is suspicious of the motives of most politicians and bemused by the thought that he may be seen to have joined their ranks. "I suspect that people may think that of me, that I have become a politician, and want to ask: What's he in it for?"

"I suspect that people may think that I have become a politician, and want to ask: What's he in it for?"

And he would reply? "My vision has not been changed, I just react differently now." He knows that he can accomplish more, for more people, on the public stage and has no plans to leave it just yet. But clinical medicine hasn't lost its appeal and he says he would be happy to go back to it. "I'll stay as long as they'll have me. But if I'm dumped, I'll go graciously."

Agnes Glaus: Softly Softly

HELEN SAUL

The President of the European Oncology Nursing Society (EONS) was having lunch with the man who was to succeed her, at a beautiful restaurant by Lake Constance in Switzerland. Suddenly serious, the President leaned forward and said, "You know, I would be so happy if EONS could have a non-smoking President." The President-Elect, a habitual smoker, promised her he would quit. And he did.

Dr Agnes Glaus, then President, is quietly influential at both a personal and professional level. Her lunch companion, Giel Vaessen, could hardly have been unaware of the dangers of smoking, and her words might have seemed patronising. But she spoke so politely and respectfully that it did not occur to him to take offence. "It was just a statement. She wasn't hectoring me. And, of course, her message was that the President of EONS is a role model and should have a healthy lifestyle. It would not be good to be seen smoking."

Reasoned argument, exquisitely delivered, often seem to get Glaus what she wants. It's a potent combination, and serves her well, whether negotiating with nurses, other health professionals, students or, increasingly, the public at large.

Glaus has devoted her career to the advancement of oncology nursing. As co-chair of the Ger-

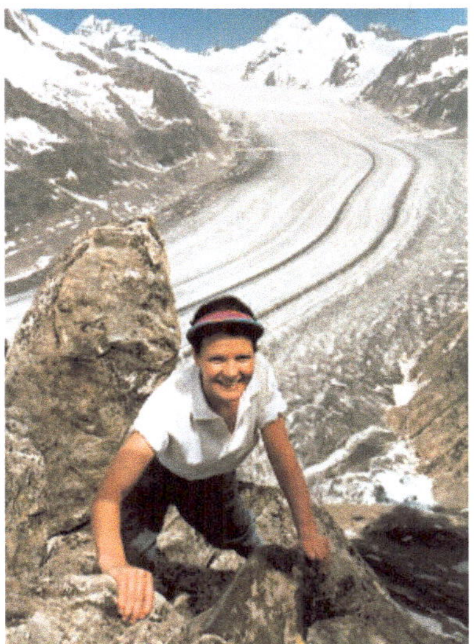

Glaus,
seen here climbing
in Switzerland,
is undaunted
by uphill struggles

man-speaking branch of European School of Oncology, she runs training courses for nurses. She has a PhD in oncology nursing and has written standard textbooks in German. And at Zentrum für Tumordiagnostik und Prävention, St Gallen, Switzerland, she combines research, teaching, prevention counselling, and cancer nursing. Plus, of course, political work at EONS.

It's a formidable workload, but one Glaus relishes. Vaessen shadowed her for the two years she was President, and his overriding impression is of a dedicated and hard worker. She copied him every email she wrote on EONS' behalf, thou-

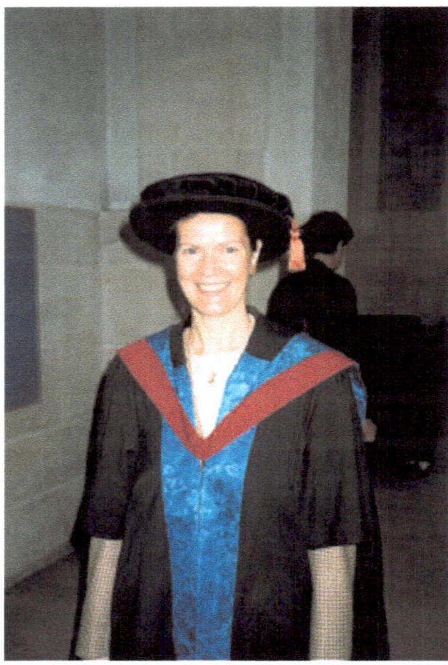

Graduation Day at the University of Surrey, where Glaus studied oncology nursing

sands and thousands in all, often sent over the weekend. Two days away from the computer, and his in-box would be full. "It would read Glaus, Glaus, Glaus, ..." he says. "Sometimes I would email back: 'Agnes, please take a rest!'".

But Glaus insisted that Vaessen needed to be informed of all EONS business. She took her role seriously and was perhaps aware that being EONS President was an important achievement not only for

Singing in the family choir

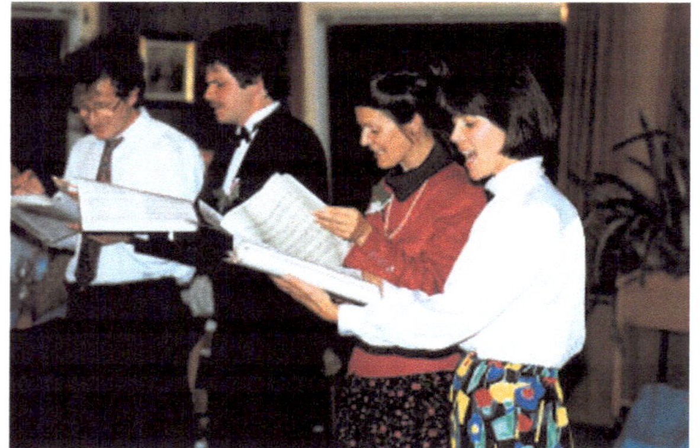

her personally. Kathy Redmond, healthcare consultant in Milan and a former EONS President, says Glaus' Presidency was a boost for German-speaking nurses throughout Europe. "It gave them, for the first time, a voice at a high level of the organisation. It's easy for us in the UK or northern Europe to become President, because we have a vision based on our experience. In the German-speaking world, oncology nursing is less developed and it is much harder. Agnes has really been the person to bring together nurses from Switzerland, Austria and Germany and to develop the art and science of oncology nursing in the German-speaking world."

Bringing people together is one of her strengths. At EONS, she was adept at getting people involved, to broaden the base of active members and share the workload. This was sometimes an uphill struggle, but Vaessen said the strain never showed. "Sometimes she would be disappointed if people would not take on a task for the society, but she was always ladylike, always polite."

"Her message was that nurses must show what we can do but must realise that we can only reach our goals in collaboration with other health professionals."

When they did respond, she made sure they knew their contribution was valued. Redmond says Glaus writes exceptional thank-you cards. "She has a wonderful way of expressing herself. Over the years her cards have made me feel really satisfied, happy and acknowledged for whatever I have done."

She worked hard for interdisciplinary collaboration. "Her message", says Vaessen, "was that nurses must show what we can do, but must realise that we can only reach our goals in collaboration with other health professionals." This attitude translated, for example, into nurses gaining access to a famous cancer training course in Switzerland, once open only to physicians. Nurses are now included in the Leonardo da Vinci accreditation scheme for health care professionals in cancer care across Europe. And, more generally, says Vaessen, she opened doors for the future for collaboration with other societies.

Collaboration is currently at risk because of a shortage of nurses throughout Europe. In her last days as President, at ECCO-11 in Lisbon, October 2001, Glaus was issuing dire warnings about the "impending danger" of the nursing shortage. "We need strong leaders to bring professions together. It is becoming increasingly difficult."

She is clearly not afraid to speak out, but neither is she a glory-seeker. EONS activated her management streak, and she devoted much of her energy as President to the low-key, even humdrum, work needed to strengthen its internal structure. Titles now have job descriptions and task lists, and officials know what is expected of them. Research projects are rigorously planned; full proposals have to be submitted, responsible people identified and all outcomes stated from the outset. Only research in keeping with the overall goals and consititution of the society is pursued. Some of her initiatives were not universally popular, but Vaessen says EONS has benefitted

from the well-defined structure and discipline she introduced.

Handing over the Presidency at ECCO was both a relief and a bit sad, she says. "It was nice, because I could see that the Society is in good shape and can grow, and I was happy to hand the everyday business over to a colleague. But it seemed very sudden and I suddenly wondered what I had done in two years! But I'm looking forward to focusing more on my own interests."

Glaus' base, at the Zentrum für Tumordiagnostik und Prävention, is in a remarkable, cylindrical building. The Zentrum takes over three of its floors and is based somewhere between a shopping centre and a local radio station. It seems an unlikely setting until you go inside. All of the rooms have huge curved windows, looking out over the outskirts of St Gallen and down to Lake Constance. Receiving chemotherapy is never going to be the high point in someone's life, but if it has to be done, it is hard to imagine a more soothing atmosphere or a better view.

Glaus loves her office. She is a co-chair and, like the physicians there, a part-owner of the non-profit-mak-

Glaus flanked by her team at the Zentrum für Tumordiagnostik und Prävention

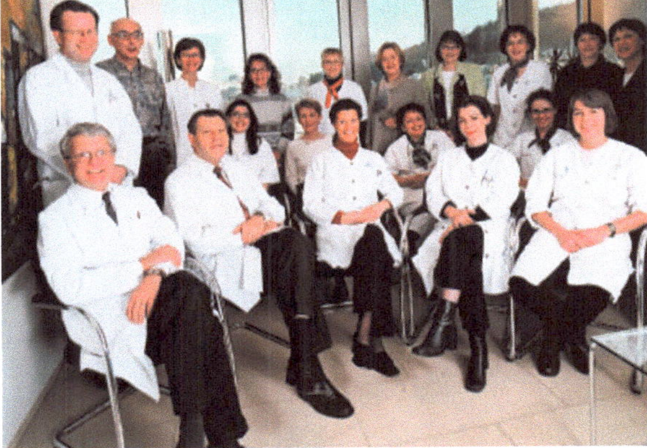

ing Zentrum. It is privately run, and care is paid for by patients' insurance companies. Research is funded by foundations. Under the leadership of Prof. Dr. Hansjörg Senn, the Zentrum opened four years ago, has steadily expanded, and now, between 120 and 150 consultations take place per week. Glaus is proud of the care on offer, which includes medical oncology, surgery, gynaecology as well as outpatient breast biopsies and, from 2002, digital mammographies. There is specialised oncology nursing care, music therapy, nutritional counselling and, of course, her own prevention counselling. The editorial offices of the Journal of Supportive Care and of Breast are also based at the centre.

All rooms look out over the outskirts of St Gallen and down to Lake Constance. It is hard to imagine a more soothing atmosphere in which to receive chemotherapy.

She has lived in this region most of her life. The Zentrum is an easy drive from the farmhouse where she grew up and where some of her family still live. Glaus was brought up as a part of a big Catholic family, she has three brothers and two sisters. One of her brothers and his family

live in the family farmhouse, along with their mother, and Glaus herself still has her own room for when she visits, which is nearly every Sunday. Her mother is 82 and needs some help. Glaus has no children of her own, which she regrets, and she takes great pleasure in her niece and four nephews.

She never wavered in her dedication to nursing. Her mother gave her a nurse's dressing-up outfit when she was very young, and she loved it. In her teens, she read Suzanna Barden's romantic books, set among nurse trainees in York, and that was it. She knew what she wanted to do.

Immediately after school, she embarked on what was then a traditional tour of Switzerland, to learn the national languages of French and Italian. She took her nursing diploma and quickly found her niche within oncology. "At first, as a student nurse working in a surgical department, I thought, 'Well, nursing is beautiful, it's heroic, this is what I want to do!' But as soon as I went into a medical department, which was more intellectual really, I knew that it was for me, and that I wouldn't be a surgical nurse after all."

"As soon as I went into a medical department, which was more intellectual really, I knew that it was for me, and that I wouldn't be a surgical nurse after all"

Glaus seems to have had a natural gift for nursing, right from the beginning. The first patient she had to nurse as a student was a woman who had undergone a mastectomy. "As a very young nurse, I didn't know how to deal with her at all, it just hap-

In China

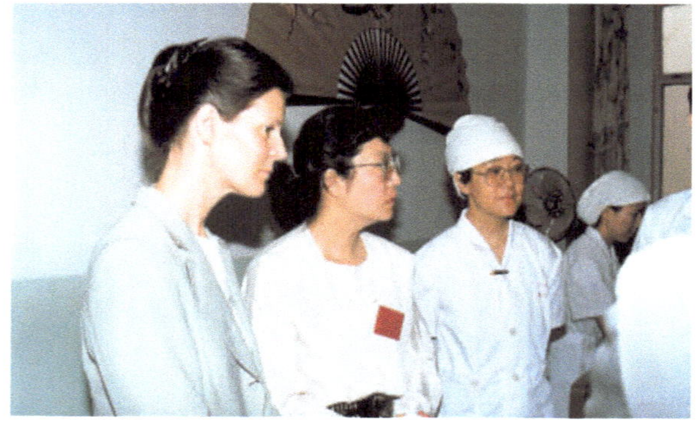

pened that I had to nurse her. But a long time after she went home, she wrote me a letter saying that the way I met her helped her so much. And I realised, at this very early stage, this is something I can do."

Her approach to people is directed by a simple Christian faith, distilled out of the Catholicism she grew up with. It can be terribly difficult when patients who have become close are desperately ill, and Glaus says that her beliefs help her deal with suffering. "It's as if I, like anyone else, am a pearl in the air, and there is a big hand below. The pearl cannot fall any further than the hand. And this is important whether I am happy or sad. I believe that I am in there, that in the end it will be fine, and that the best is still to come."

"Being with a patient is the main inspiration for research. I'm always thinking: What is she telling me in relation to what I have read? Does it fit with my theoretical ideas?"

Her special talent lies in her respect for patients and her willingness to take on board their point of view, even where it contradicts accepted wisdom. This has also given her the starting point for research. "When I'm sitting in front of a patient and we're talking, I think: 'What is she telling me in relation to what I have read, or written? Does it fit with my theoretical ideas?' Being with patients is the main inspiration for research."

Research has become an important part of her work. Glaus has a Master's degree and a doctorate in oncology nursing, both from the University of Surrey, UK. Her mentor

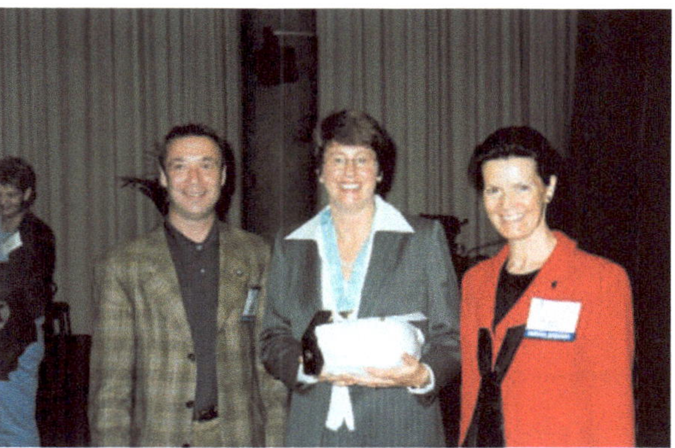

there was Prof. Rosemary Crow, who is now retired. "She had an elaborate and sophisticated understanding of what nursing is, and what science is. She liked good scientific work and interdisciplinary work," says Glaus. "She supported scientific work in an interdisciplinary environment. She never compromised the independence of nursing, but she believed it was at its strongest as part of an interdisciplinary team. She had a great influence on me."

These principles have guided Glaus throughout. She went on, as part of her PhD, to learn the qualitative methodologies particularly suited to many nursing topics. They include in-depth interviews and content analysis, and can be very sound science, but are often not well understood by other professionals. Undeterred, she has continued to carry out nursing research, stressing that it is complementary to the mostly quantitative work done by physicians.

Her long-standing interest in fatigue among cancer patients started during her Master's degree when, in the early 1990s, she set out to examine patients' problems. "In this piece of research, fatigue was the most im-

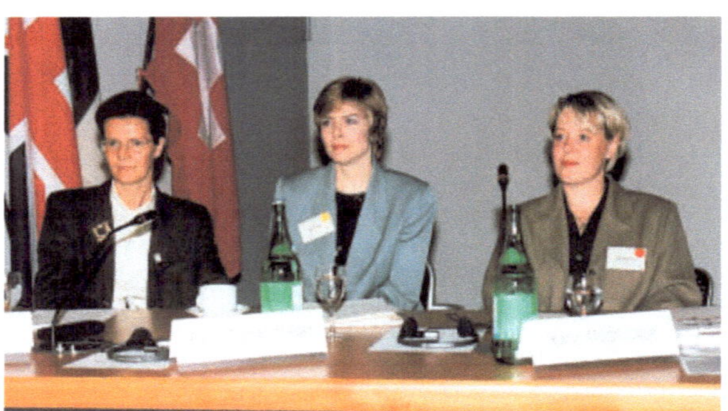

Glaus enjoys the international dimension. Here, with the Presidents of American and Swedish Oncology Nursing Societies

portant problem. It was surprising and impressive; we hadn't considered it before. When I searched the literature, I found colleagues in the States had started to research it. But only since then has fatigue become a discussed scientific issue.

"Fatigue is the most frequent and distressing symptom, but care-givers do not communicate well on the subject. Patients think that we are not interested, or can do nothing."

"Even now, though, people are not sufficiently aware of the problem. Fatigue is the most frequent and distressing symptom of most cancer patients, but physicians and nurses do not communicate well on the subject. Patients do not feel properly understood. They think either that fatigue is of no interest to their care-givers, or that nothing can be done to help. We have just held a research focus group with patients and they told us that they are desperate to talk about fatigue, and to have their symptoms – which nobody sees or can understand – taken seriously."

At present, she is most enthusiastic about an EONS research project on nausea and emesis. She set it up while President, and is still co-or-dinator. It is being conducted with an industrial partner, and preliminary results will be reported at the EONS Spring Convention in Venice. What's exciting her is that the project involves collaboration with nurses from Germany, Austria, Spain, and Switzerland. "In German-speaking regions, nurses are not usually involved in research. It was so nice to find colleagues full of energy and enthusiasm for research, and just to help them grasp what they need to grasp to do this research. Collaborative nursing research across different European countries is a new area. Many nurses are involved in medical research and work as part of a medical team. But this is a nursing project, based on nursing practice and run by nurses. It was so nice to see colleagues in Germany and Austria being so well accepted by their medical colleagues. It was a highlight of my time as President."

Another new and expanding avenue for her is in prevention counselling, usually for relatives of patients at the Zentrum. But she'd like eventually to offer the service to the women shopping, just a few floors below. Already, she gives talks to women's groups, mother and toddler groups, groups at gyms. "It's a favourite of mine, going to speak to lay populations. I like it very much. They are so interested and they learn so much. Sometimes at professional organisations, people are either sceptical or not very interested."

"The paradigm of our times is cure. But molecular biology has made it a good time to reflect: Isn't there a better way? Shouldn't we be better at preventing tumours?"

She believes that prevention is a subject whose time has, belatedly, come. "The paradigm of our times is cure; we focus on destroying the disease, even though we can cure only a small proportion of our patients. But prevention demands a special understanding of health and trying to support or regain health is different from destroying disease. New knowledge of the molecular biological background of tumours, and influences from our surroundings, have made it a good time to reflect: Isn't there a better way? Shouldn't we be better at preventing tumours or detecting them early? Prevention has always made sense, but it has taken us a long time to focus on it."

Glaus says she will also be taking on more university-level teaching, and she's aiming to make more time for her many neglected interests. She has sung since she was a young girl in the church choir with her brothers and sisters, and she's intending to join another choir. Then there's pottery; she has a love of art, of forms and shapes. And of nature, walking in the mountains, in forests, and by the lake, all so close to St Gallen. And perhaps a little more time off, though she says that even at her busiest, it can sometimes only take a day to recover. Once, after lecturing in Milan, she and a friend climbed to the top of the Cathedral tower. "It was such a beautiful day. The colours were light, the sky was blue and standing outside for two hours at the top of the dome was worth a week's holiday. I took home intense feelings, of art and nature and light and friendship. And a beautiful experience like this is far more important for me, than having a long holiday."

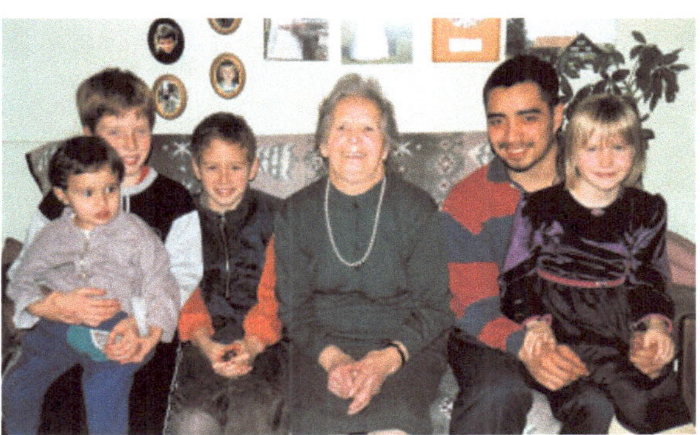

There's no sign of a decreasing workload for Glaus, and she acknowledges that not having children has contributed to her drive. "It would have been the most wonderful thing, but it just didn't happen. It is a sorrow, but an accepted sorrow.

"I have been able to pass on knowledge to many nurses, and maybe this is a way of creating new generations"

"The other side of it is that I have been able to pass on knowledge to many nurses, and maybe this is a way of creating new generations, which is very important. Prevention work also is for the future. What we do today will be the future."

In fact, Vaessen says he sometimes thinks of her in the role of mother or teacher. As President-elect, he learned a terrific amount from her, and in his first months as President is still influenced by her. "It's weird. I'm writing reports for the society on our goals and future aims at the moment, and I can hear her voice. She's saying: 'Please think of this, or that.' And I say: 'Yes, mum!' I don't always agree with her, but I'm always interested in her opinion."

Glaus comes from a large Catholic family. Here her mother poses with her nephews and neice

Mariano Barbacid: The Homecoming

HELEN SAUL

The view from the balcony of Prof. Mariano Barbacid's office stretches out over the northern suburbs of Madrid, right down to the centre of the city itself. In the foreground, at what was the northern edge of the city only a few decades ago, is the apartment block where he lived as a child.

It sounds cosy, parochial even, to be able to see someone's birthplace from their office. It's a false impression. Barbacid's career has been played out on the big stage. He took initial degrees in Madrid, certainly, but then spent 24 glittering years in the US, which included discovering the first human oncogene. He returned in 1998, with a brief to build Spain its first big cancer research centre, from scratch.

Barbacid intends the new research centre to be on a level with similar major insitutions anywhere in the world. It is an uphill task. Spain has little tradition in basic research, and it will take time to find staff of sufficient calibre who are keen to work in Madrid. Even the public is bemused by the undertaking. "Spaniards are very much into the humanities, but have no interest in research," says Barbacid. "It's a matter of culture. We have sensibility for poetry, and understand its importance beyond the needs of our daily lives. But we have none of that feeling for research."

This is changing, in part because of Spain's strengthening economy. In the past 25 years, the health system has improved dramatically, and is now as good as the European Union average. But research still has a low priority.

"Spaniards have sensibility for poetry, and understand its importance beyond the needs of our daily lives. But we have none of that feeling for research."

In 1996, Dr. José Antonio Gutiérrez Fuentes, a former cardiologist who left medicine for politics, came to a position of power. He recognised the need for research cen-

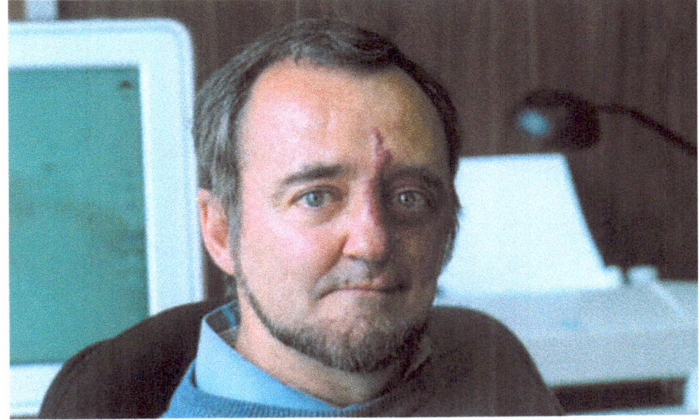

tres for the diseases that kill most Spaniards: cancer, cardiovascular and neurodegenerative diseases. He contacted Barbacid and asked him to shoulder responsibility for the Centro Nacional de Investigaciones Oncológicas (CNIO) – the Spanish National Cancer Centre. They agreed on budget, size of operation, management structure, and so on, and in 1998 Barbacid came back to Spain and took on, he says, "a real challenge".

First, there was the renovation of an existing hospital, the old Victoria Eugenia, a hospital located within the campus of the Instituto de Salud Carlos III that had been closed for more than 15 years, and a whole new block to put up. Building started in August 1999, and Barbacid moved into his new office in February 2002. Speedy work, especially at a time when demand for construction was at almost unprecedented levels – some say that building was one of few outlets for undeclared pesetas, and demand soared before the introduction of the Euro.

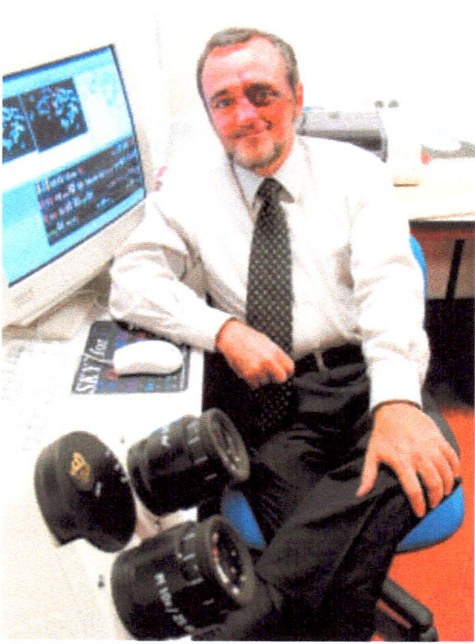

Whatever. By 2006, the CNIO will house 400 professionals. The Spanish government will pay up to 60 percent of the running costs, but it is managed like a private institution. Barbacid can implement his own ideas, programmes and initiatives, and take on the department heads he wants. They in turn are given a free hand – with the caveat, of course, that if it all goes wrong, those given responsibility take the rap. None of this sounds extraordinary, but it is rare in Spain. Directors of other research centres have little power to hire and fire, since their senior scientific staff are civil servants and remain in position no matter what they do. Barbacid: "When you know somebody is watching you and that you are being constantly reviewed and checked, you tend to do things much better than if you know nothing will ever happen to you, no matter how poor your performance. It's just human nature."

At CNIO, the basic research programme will cover molecular oncology, cancer genetics, structural biology and biocomputing. The applied research programmes will include molecular pathology, experimental therapeutics, biotechnology and medicinal chemistry. CNIO will house the Spanish National Tumour Bank network and investigate hereditary cancer. Barbacid's own laboratory is part of molecular oncology, but he sees the combination of basic and applied research as crucial to the institute's success: "In cancer we have just come through a golden age of accumulating knowledge. Now the challenge is to apply the knowledge."

Barbacid's dream, now, is for himself and his staff at CNIO to find another drug – like Glivec – that is designed to block a specific molecular target. It is ambitious, but not impossible. In his own career, Barbacid has always played to his strengths. Now that a whole institute is arranged along such lines, who knows what could happen?

Barbacid's dream, now, is for himself and his staff at CNIO to find another drug – like Glivec – that is designed to block a specific molecular target

Barbacid himself was born in Madrid and, like many other teenage boys, was attracted to science by the big questions about the Big Bang and the origin of matter. Realising that he did not particularly excel at mathematics, though, he switched his focus and took his first degree in chemistry at the University of Madrid. He found straight chemistry rather dry, so added a biological component, and took his MSc and PhD in biochemistry, again in Madrid.

He does not remember why he chose cancer, except that it was a challenge and, at the time, retroviruses were creating excitement. In 1974, he left Spain for the laboratory of RNA Tumor Viruses at the National Cancer Institute in the US. A good move.

He does not remember why he chose cancer, except that it was a challenge, and at the time, retroviruses were creating excitement.

Before 1970, it had been known that carcinogens such as tobacco cause cancer, but the mechanism was still a mystery. A tiny retrovirus, which causes cancer in chickens, was to yield important clues. The virus is much less potent when grown in culture, and scientists found that it lost 1000 of its 9000 nucleotides there. Further, the lost nucleotides alone cause cancer when injected into chickens. Crucially, the retroviral sequence was then found to originate from normal chicken cells. It had been modified to become cancer causing.

"That's the moment I arrived in the States," said Barbacid. "I was very fortunate in terms of timing. It was almost at the beginning of the molecular biology of cancer."

After completing his postdoc at NCI, Barbacid was offered his own lab there by Dr. Stuart Aaronson. Aaronson also handed over part of his own research for Barbacid to work on independently. It convinced Barbacid to stay in the US, even though he had just been offered an associate professorship at a Spanish university. "That turned out to be one of the critical decisions in my life," he says now. "I decided not only to continue with this line of research, but I inherited a gift, which allowed me to develop my own line of research. Then something very fortunate happened."

A friend was working at Columbia with Richard Axel and Mike Wiggler on transferring DNA into cells in culture, a major achievement at the time. The assay was based on a cell line deficient in thymidine kinase. They transferred DNA, including the gene that codes for the enzyme. The cells then grew, and it had to be because the DNA had been incorporated.

"I was very fortunate in terms of timing. It was almost at the beginning of the molecular biology of cancer."

Barbacid argued that if tumours, like viruses, had oncogenes, they should be detected by the same technique. He spent a weekend with his friend, learned the technique, and came back and started using it. What he and his lab – himself, two post-docs and a technician – needed to show was that the oncogene came from human cells. "Sequencing is now no big deal, but in those days it was not so clear that what we were finding in transformed cells was a gene. We really had to isolate it."

A prohibition on cloning in the US had been lifted only a couple of years previously, and the technology was in its infancy. But the race to find the first human oncogene was on. Within a few months, it was apparently over. One of Barbacid's post-docs, Eugenio Santos, came into the laboratory in the summer of 1981, looking rather dejected and waving a copy of the New York Times. Bob Weinberg at MIT, and the same Mike Wiggler, by then at Cold Spring Harbor, had cloned the first human oncogene, it said. Beaten, and they had only just started.

Barbacid, ever pragmatic, insisted the research continue. If his lab was to continue with the project, they would still have to clone the gene. Even if they had been beaten over the first hurdle, other lines of investigation would still be open to them.

It was a good decision. Not only had the New York Times got the story wrong – nobody had cloned the gene at that stage – but the article focussed attention on Weinberg and Wiggler, who were consequently inundated with invitations to talk. Out of the spotlight, Barbacid's team worked on: "We didn't get distracted. Even though there were only four of us, we were able to catch up."

"Nature called 1982 the Year of the Oncogene. It was my best year, we got three editorials."

In the end, all three groups isolated the gene at the same time. Wiggler published at the end of April 1982 in Nature; Barbacid in PNAS (Proceedings of the National Academy of Sciences) and Weinberg in Cell in May 1982. Barbacid then demonstrated that the human oncogene was from the ras family of genes, previously isolated from

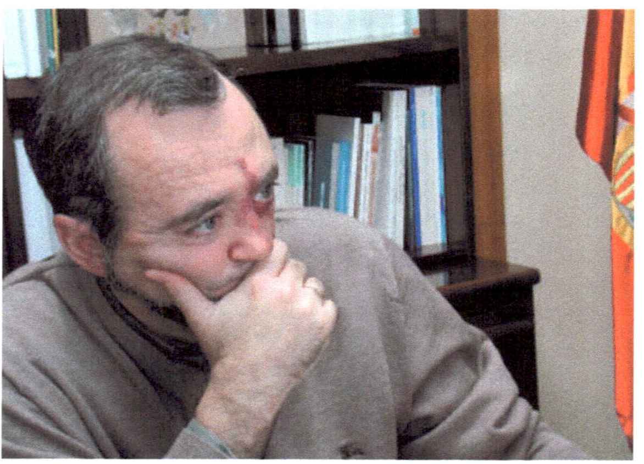

rodent retroviruses. He discovered that the oncogene differed from the normal gene only in a single point mutation, and showed that the oncogenes were frequently activated not only in tumour cell lines, but in cancer patients. This was published in Nature later the same year, back to back with Weinberg's work on the mechanism of action. In 1984, Barbacid, in collaboration with scientists from the Istituto di Tumori in Milan, identified a mutated ras oncogene in the lung adenocarcinoma of a patient, but not in his normal tissue, demonstrating at the same time the somatic nature of cancer mutations.

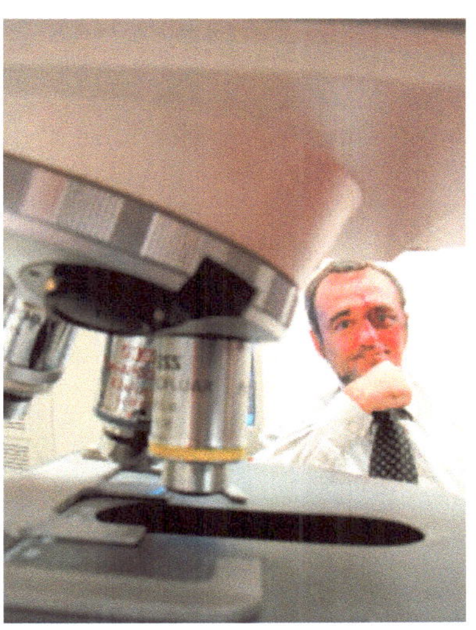

Barbacid: "Nature called 1982 the Year of the Oncogene. It was my best year, we got three editorials in Nature. It may have been a bit overstated, some people thought there was too much excitement. Obviously, it was an important step, but it was just one step."

From there, the molecular biology of human cancer took off. In 1983, chromosomal translocations were shown to alter expression levels of genes originally found in retroviruses. Soon afterwards came the discovery of tumour suppressor genes, and progress accelerated.

Barbacid's contribution was recognised by a clutch of awards from both Spain and the US, and the discovery set the pattern for his next few years.

Barbacid's contribution was recognised by a clutch of awards from both Spain and the US, and the discovery set the pattern for his next few years. He used animal models to show that the oncogenes are the targets of chemical carcinogens. The model system was used to establish that activation of ras oncogenes is one of the earliest events in the development of tumours. He then went on to discover other human oncogenes, in particular trk and vav, which have had a major impact in the research community.

So by the time he was 38 years old, Barbacid had an impressive track record at NIH. He was happily supervising 12 people, but could see that he had reached his ceiling. He was approached by Squibb, which had been a small pharmaceutical company until scientists at the company developed the first ACE inhibitor through rational design. Squibb suddenly had a lot of money, and wanted to invest in research. Barbacid joined the company to build a department of molecular biology, with no commitment to drug discovery.

A couple of years later, Bristol Myers bought Squibb. Barbacid: "Science was no longer the driving force, and I realised there would be no future for me at the company without doing drug discovery. To begin with, that's why I started it – it was a survival instinct. But I came to enjoy it, because after a while, publishing paper after paper, discovering oncogenes or finding that this phosphorylates that, was not totally fulfilling for me. When you have the means to discover molecules that cure cancer – unfortunately only in mice – but still cure cancer, this is something else. The high, the excitement, is comparable to what I felt in 1981."

"When you have the means to discover molecules that cure cancer – unfortunately only in mice – but still cure cancer, this is something else."

It was new territory for Barbacid, as was the training he received in business and management. He ran a department of 125, and was part of an organisation of 1000. "It meant planning strategically and meeting goals – not something scientists usu-ally bother with. I learnt a lot which I value now."

Barbacid remained at the company for almost nine years, initiating and supervising drug discovery programmes in, among other areas, cytotoxics, oncogenes and tumour suppressor genes, angiogenesis inhibitors and apoptosis. Alongside this work, he was able to continue a basic research programme, until March 1997, when a change in upper management led to its cancellation and forced Barbacid out. He was preparing to go to MD Anderson (Houston, Texas) when he was approached by Gutiérrez Fuentes. "I would have said no if he had contacted me a year earlier or a year later. Perhaps it was the right time. I realised that whatever I built at MD Anderson, even if I was successful, it would be one out of 100 in the States. Coming back to Spain, it is one out of one. So perhaps that is why I decided to come back, coupled with the fact that I'm Spanish and somehow you always want to go back to your roots."

"I grew up in a fascist dictatorship and have a fairly developed sense of social justice. The US is a system of perfect social justice if you forget the lower 25%."

He enjoyed living in the US, and remains thankful for the way he was treated there. "But I grew up in a fascist dictatorship and have a fairly developed sense of social justice. The US is a system of perfect social justice if you forget the lower 25%. They don't have health insurance, they go to schools where they don't even learn to read. I'm a totally con-

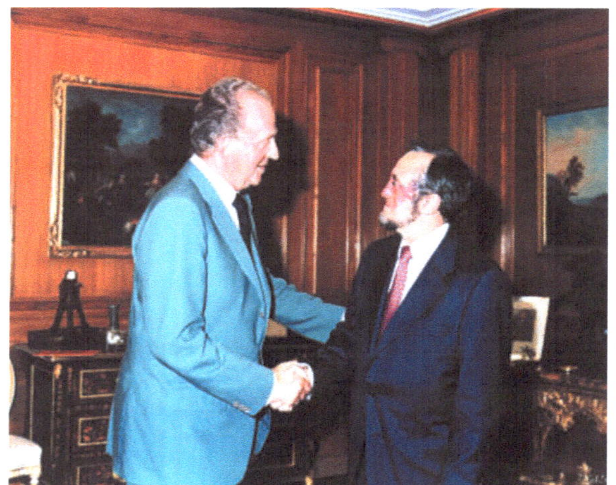

Barbacid with Juan Carlos I, the King of Spain

vinced European and found it hard to think I was a part of that system."

Family was no obstacle to his return. Barbacid had been previously married to an American, but at the time of Gutiérrez Fuentes' offer, was dating a Spaniard, Monica. They came back together, got married in 1999, and now have a toddler, Carmen. Fatherhood has cut down on his travelling and reduced his working week from 70 to a mere 60 hours, as he goes home at 8.15 pm every evening to bathe and play with his daughter. He enjoys good food, particularly oriental food, and loves symphonic and chamber music. He says he became addicted to opera while working at Princeton for Bristol Myers Squibb, but has never learned to play. "I have a terrible ear, I can not reproduce a note. It's very frustrating but that's the way it is."

"If I led you to climb through a simple pile of dirt, and then declared you ready to climb Everest, you would probably die in the attempt. Preclinical assays are too simple."

He remains inspired by his number one hobby: work. His current research project is to improve preclinical screening of compounds. There are more than 300 compounds in clinical trials in cancer around the world, of which only a handful will be approved. The success rate is dismal. Preclinical models are not adequately predicting clinical outcome, he argues. "If I led you to climb through a simple pile of dirt, and then declared you ready to climb Everest, you would probably die in the attempt. Preclinical assays are too

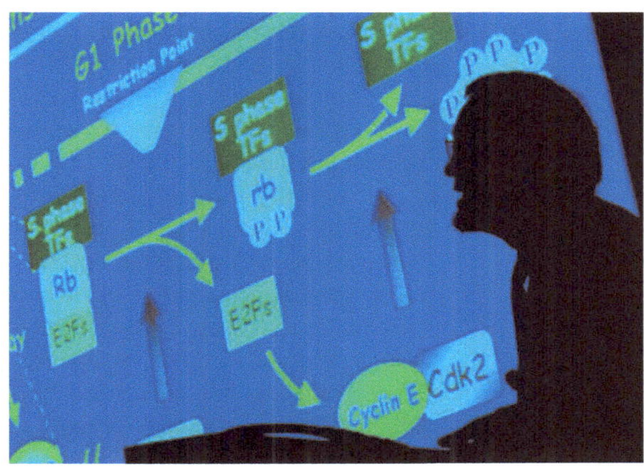

simple. Too many compounds are getting through and then failing in the real world."

Barbacid's lab is manipulating mice embryos to make mice with the same genetic mutations that cause cancer in humans. Tumours are still of mouse origin, so the system is not perfect, but tumour characteristics and physiology are closely related to human cancers. This type of work is being carried out in only a handful of centres around the world, but Barbacid wants CNIO in the top league.

The institute is one of the first in Europe to have its own microarray technology to facilitate basic research. Another department will take on drug discovery. "We do not intend to compete with the major pharmaceutical companies, but we're not under the same business pressure as they are, and we think we could do something. They work with 20, 30 or 50 targets. We will select one or two. And if we find a drug candidate, it will be ours. We will never be able to do full development, but at least we can license it and that will give us enough money to pay for our operations. I'm daydreaming maybe, but we are going to give it a shot."

It's a tall order, but given Barbacid's professional history, it would be brave to bet against him.

He sees the story of Glivec as the model to follow. Ciba Geigy, now Novartis, set out to target the easiest molecule in cancer. Barbacid and two scientists from Dana Farber were taken on as advisors in 1986. They suggested the oncogene bcr-abl, which only appears in chronic myeloid leukaemia. CML does not mean big business like some other cancers, but the company pursued this line for 15 years, and in the end succeeded.

Barbacid is clear about his approach: "We should not think in business terms, we should think that in cancer, you never know where

"We won't care whether the targets we choose will cure lung cancer, which is the biggest killer, or breast cancer which has the biggest incidence. We are going to go conceptually."

you are going to find the next molecule. I'm taking that lesson here. We won't care whether the targets we choose will cure lung cancer, which is the biggest killer, or breast cancer which has the biggest incidence. We are going to go conceptually. That is a luxury we have that pharmaceutical companies don't, or at least only a few dare to take. We hope that will give us some advantage, and that we'll get a result before I retire or die, which will probably happen on the same day. I hope to live long enough to see it."

Liisa Elovainio: Tough on Tobacco

HELEN SAUL

Dr. Liisa Elovainio almost burst into tears when she met the Pope. Not because it was a meaningful religious experience (she is not a Catholic), nor because she was overcome by the event. Rather, it was because the cardinal introducing her had just announced to a rapt audience of 40,000 people at St Peter's Square that cancer research and treatment are important. His Holiness the Pope was pleased to learn that the Association of European Cancer Leagues had been discussing ethical issues at a cancer conference in Rome.

Liisa Elovainio has devoted her professional life to the fight against cancer and against tobacco, playing a leading role in campaigns that changed Finland from a country with the highest smoking rates in the world, to one with the among lowest tobacco consumption in Europe. In recognition of her contribution, she was made a Knight, First Class, of the Order of the Lion of Finland, in 1985. She has been Secretary General of the Cancer Society of Finland since 1987, and is chair of the board of the Finnish Centre for Health Education. Elovainio gained international recognition when she was awarded the Cancer Control Bronze Medal by the Cancer Society of Finland in 1997 and the WHO Tobacco Control Medal in 1999. She's been a member of the council of the International Union Against Cancer (UICC) since 1988 and has held one of the top positions in the Association of European Cancer Leagues (ECL) since 1996. She is currently immersed in organising the 12th World Conference on Tobacco or Health: Global Action for a Tobacco-Free Future, to be held in her home town of Helsinki in 2003. As President of the Conference, she wants it to be special, and is concentrating on ensuring the funds are there to enable a strong participation from the developing world and Eastern Europe, which are now on the front line of tobacco industry marketing.

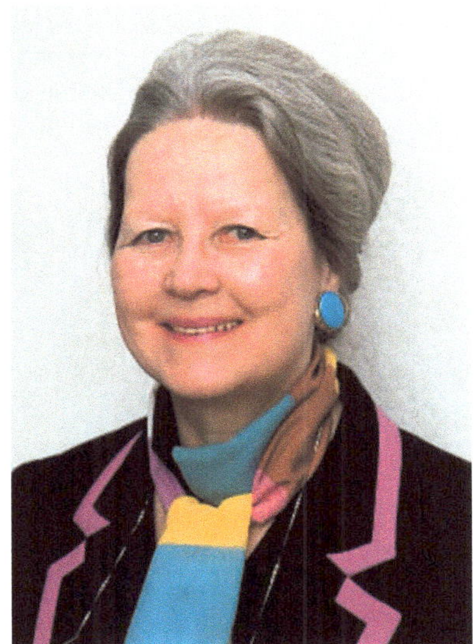

In the end, she retained her composure, but, characteristically, her joy in the occasion lay in the unexpected opportunity to spread the cancer message. A personal compliment from one of the most influential men on earth was somewhat incidental.

Elovainio, then President of the Association of European Cancer Leagues (ECL), has been Secretary General of the Cancer Society of Finland since 1987. She was its Chief of Health Education for the previous 12 years and has just been re-elected to the Council of the International Union Against Cancer (UICC). At both national and international levels, she has been a key player in the drive to reduce the burden of cancer, in particular through improved screening and tobacco control.

The Finnish experience, with Elovainio at the helm, has become a role model for the rest of Europe. Cigarette consumption, which was the highest in the world in the 1920s, is now among the lowest in Europe. It's a meaningful reduction, as lung cancer rates have followed the same downward curve. Cancer screening programmes achieve remarkable participation rates: 70% in a current colorectal screening pilot, and the same in a prostate cancer screening study. In breast cancer screening, 88% of women respond to invitations. "This is an obedient population. It is almost as if they think something terrible will happen if they don't come," she says.

When the incidence of cervical cancer started to rise, epidemiologists established that participation in screening had declined. The Society revamped its efforts to get women to come forward, and the incidence leveled off.

But it's also a population that has been well served by its Cancer Society over many years. The Cancer Society is independent and non-political. It incorporates the Finnish Cancer Foundation, Finnish Cancer Registry and the Finnish Foundation for Cancer Research. This means that more than half of the staff at its headquarters are researchers, mostly epidemiologists. Prevention strategies are devised in-house; facts on publicity material can be checked on the spot. When worrying trends appear in the data, the whole Society is alerted and consulted. In the mid-1990s, for example, the incidence of cervical cancer, which had been falling, started to rise. Epidemiologists established that this was a result of declining participation in screening in the big cities. The Society revamped its efforts to get women to come forward, and the incidence leveled off again.

The Cancer Society sets the agenda for screening in Finland and conducts most cervical and breast cancer screening throughout the

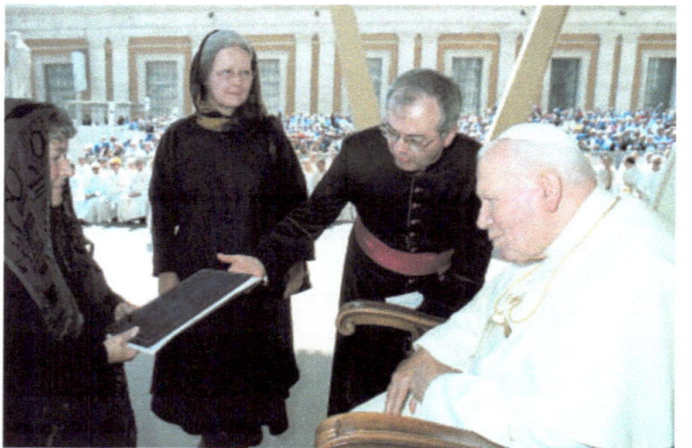

September 2000. Mrs Lilly Christensen, ECL President (far left) and Dr. Elovainio are introduced to the Pope

country. Health promotion is another priority, as is the establishment of screening for other cancers.

A national study into colorectal cancer screening, based on an improved haemoccult test, is also being set up. It aims to determine the cost of screening and the frequency of false-positives and -negatives. In prostate cancer, Finland is part of the pan-European screening pilot, set up 4 years ago against a background of enormous pressure within Europe for PSA (prostate specific antigen) screening tests to become routine. So far, the pilot has established that early cancers are being detected. "Even so, we don't know whether we are doing more harm than good. We have to wait a few more years for mortality comparisons between those who participated and those who received an invitation but didn't turn up for screening," says Elovainio.

Elovainio takes great pride in the quality of the existing screening programmes and the reliability of the data on which they are based. The Cancer Registry is owned by the Society and is housed on the floor above her office. It holds data on every patient in the country, with the many notifications for each patient making the records highly reliable. When doubts about screening are raised in the international community, such as the recent furore over the value of mammography, the Finns instinctively turn to and trust their own data. In Finland, mammography is carried out throughout the country and not concentrated in a few centres of excellence. Even so, it appears to reduce breast cancer mortality in the country by almost 30%. End of debate.

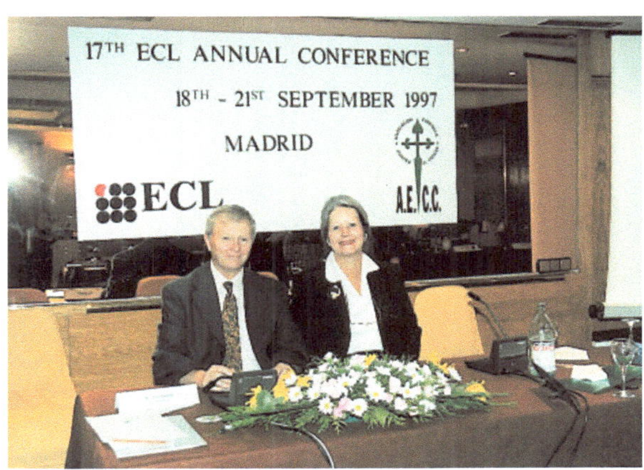

Screening in Finland is a source of quiet satisfaction for Elovainio. She was Secretary General at the Cancer Society when the mammography programme was set up. "It is like my baby somehow," she says. The Cancer Society does of course have to raise the funds to carry out its activities, but it runs smoothly, quality is monitored rigorously, procedures followed and patients looked after. Upsets are rare.

The same cannot be said for the tobacco reduction programme. Upsets here are routine, but Elovainio obviously relishes the fight. It is psychological warfare. She has been involved in numerous campaigns, conferences and debates over the years and is intensely aware of the pervasive influence of the industry. "Every so often the tobacco industry weighs into a debate disguised as the 'Foundation for Socially Responsible Behaviour' or some such title. So at first you don't realise that it's a tobacco industry organisation. But somebody somewhere in Europe will know, and will immediately pass the information on through our European networks, warning everyone else."

With Tom Hudson from Dublin (immediate past president of the ECL)

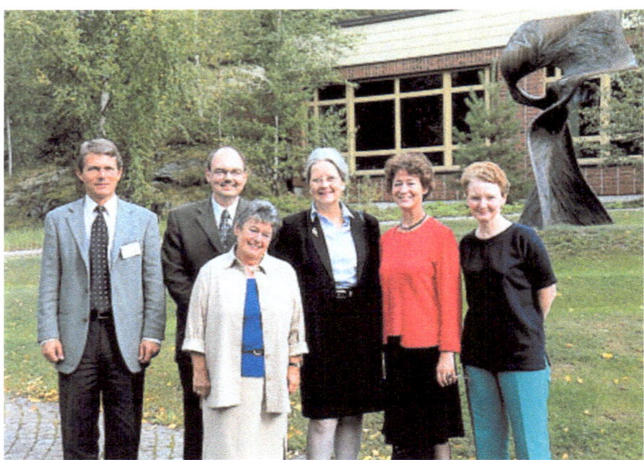

Secretary Generals of the Nordic Cancer Union (NCU), pictured at the joint NCU-ANCR (Association of Nordic Cancer Registries) symposium in Helsinki September 2001
Left to right:
Thomas Moeller Thomsen (Secretary General, Danish Cancer Society) Jákup N. Olsen (Chairman, Faroese Association Against Cancer) Lilly Christensen (Secretary General, Norwegian Cancer Society)Liisa Elovainio (Secretary General, Cancer Society of Finland) Gudrún Agnarsdóttir (Director, Icelandic Cancer Society) Marianne af Malmborg (Secretary General, Swedish Cancer Society)

Every day she devotes some time to reducing smoking, either at national or international levels. "This is the most important thing I can ever imagine in cancer control," she says.

In the early years, civil liberty arguments held sway, with the industry saying it was entitled to freedom of speech and that, in any case, advertising does not increase smoking. Elovainio was exasperated. "Everywhere else, advertising increases consumption, but they claimed it was not true for smoking. It was totally illogical, but the media wanted the money from the advertisements and so they didn't question it."

Other industry tactics, she argues, are pernicious. Columnists and academics are paid to include pro-tobacco arguments in newspapers, magazines and even journals. Delegates are planted at conferences and attempt to sway discussions in the industry's favour, or at least to deflect attention on to obesity or some other health problem. Further, the industry funds research into cancer. Elovainio cannot understand researchers accepting this money. "The whole point of their work is to diminish suffering from cancer. So why would they take this money and allow the industry to improve its image? It is not logical. We do not give money to those whom we know are accepting money from the tobacco industry."

"The tobacco industry might weigh into a debate disguised as the 'Foundation for Socially Responsible Behaviour'. But somebody somewhere in Europe will know it is an industry organisation, and will immediately warn everyone else."

Some years ago, Elovainio found herself subject to personal ridicule in the lay press, accused of exaggeration and being paranoid about the intentions of the industry. Her opponent in the debate was an eloquent spokesman for the tobacco industry, whose phrases were so humourous and well put that they were quoted at length. She had to reply, to get the opposite case across, but criticism was directed at her rather than her arguments, and it was bruising. Now, she shrugs at the memory and says only that she had good friends who kept phoning to ask how she was tolerating it all. "That was nice," she says.

Personal ridicule is one of the industry tactics revealed in the papers made available after the success of the court cases in the US. These papers have been critically important, Elovainio says. "Many times we thought we knew what the industry was up to, but we couldn't prove it. Now we have data on their ruthless behaviour."

Some aspects of smoking behaviour are so complicated that some of the least helpful suggestions come from those who are genuinely trying to help. At present, reduction of smoking among young people is a priority. How to achieve this aim is another matter. Elovainio is a member of the Finnish delegation to the World Health Organisation's Framework Convention on Tobacco or Health. "Even some people from very progressive countries thought it would be a good thing to print across cigarette packets: Not to be sold to people under 18 years old. This is a dream for the tobacco industry, because it is likely to make smoking even more attractive to youngsters. They want to take risks, they want to show their friends how tough they are; they are 12 years old, but they can buy a packet of cigarettes with this warning on. You can assume it would be counterproductive.

"The tobacco industry never opposes campaigns directed at young people. From this you can conclude that that they are ineffective in reducing smoking."

Current Finnish campaigns give out tough messages about death. Extensive interviews with Finnish teenagers have established that they think frightening messages are the most effective, though sentiment on this matter has fluctuated over the years, and sometimes campaigns have had to be only soft and encouraging. "At the moment, it's quite the opposite and the message is really tough," says Elovainio.

Initially it appears to be some sort of a horror movie, with its black and red introduction, and unnerving statements such as "When death comes, you're alone."

For example, an interactive website has been constructed under the name "Serial Killer" (www.serialkiller.fi). Initially it appears to be some sort of a horror movie, with its black and red introduction, and unnerving statements such as "When death comes, you're alone". In fact, it contains stories, fact sheets and video clips; and it becomes apparent only gradually that the site is about tobacco and the harm it causes. Users have to figure this out for themselves. One part of the site includes an addiction test and the "profiler", which asks users how many ciga-

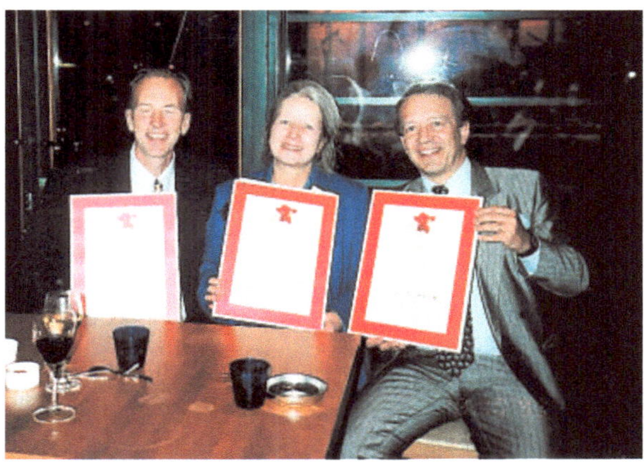

Receiving the WHO Tobacco-Free World Award for her outstanding contribution to public health, 31 May 1999. With Pekka Puska (right) and Olaf Fagerström (left)

rettes they smoke, their age and the year they started smoking. It then calculates the total number of cigarettes smoked and the amount of money spent on cigarettes, the number of trees cut down as a result, and the number of days of life lost because of smoking. This part of the programme is also available via mobile phones. Users send in their data in a text message and receive the results the same way.

But however imaginative such campaigns are, Elovainio maintains that the key to reducing smoking lies with the Government "Without legislation, it is just Sunday talk, a nice campaign here and there, the occasional good slogan, but no long-term effect. To be effective, you must be backed up with legislation and price policy." she says.

> **"Without legislation [on tobacco control], it is just Sunday talk, a nice campaign here and there, but no long term effect. To be effective, you must be backed up with legislation and price policy."**

Finland now has some of the toughest legislation in the world. The progressive Measures for the Restriction of Tobacco Smoking Act was passed in 1976, and included a total advertising ban, prohibition of sale of tobacco products to minors, and prohibition of smoking in public premises and on most public transport. The Act was tightened in 1995 to protect employees from environmental tobacco smoke, and to prohibit indirect tobacco advertising and sponsoring. In 1999, a further law ensured that all but the smallest restaurants have a smoke-free area.

Elovainio's job, then, covers a wide area. She negotiates with the Government on matters of health promotion, working with Dr. Matti Rautalahti, the current health promotion Chief at the Cancer Society, to devise campaigns with the best possible chance of success. She oversees research and fundraising at the Cancer Society. And she also has strong international ties through her work at both the Association of European Cancer Leagues and the International Union Against Cancer.

> **"As a hospital psychologist, I saw that the doctors took all the decisions, even if I knew better" Elovainio went back to university and re-trained in medicine.**

She is strangely well qualified for her job. She entered university to study French and English, but switched to sociology and completed her degree. She was interested in medical sociology and became a hospital psychologist. "Then I saw that the doctors took all the decisions, even if I knew better as a psychologist." Elovainio went back to univer-

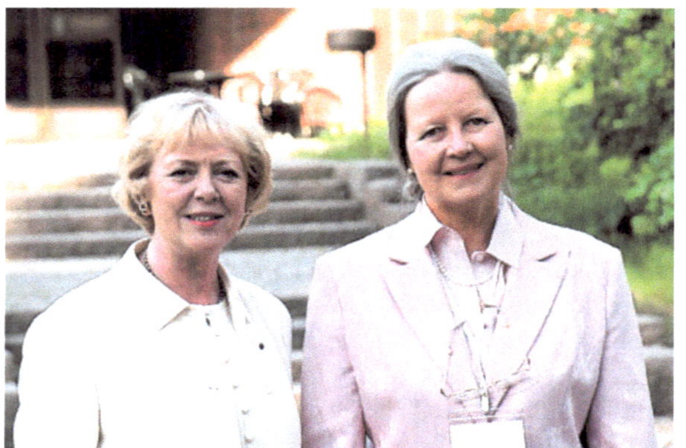

sity at the age of 25 and re-trained as a doctor.

In one way or another, she has moved in international circles all her life. She was born just before the outbreak of the Second World War, in a small town on the west coast of Finland. A few months later, the family moved to within 12 kilometres of the Russian border. Her father was a lung specialist, and the whole family lived in the tuberculosis hospitals where he worked. Russian prisoners of war worked in the hospital garden, guarding it from hungry Finnish doctors wanting a few extra vegetables. In fact, one of her earliest memories is of playing 100 metres away from home and watching a parachutist descend right in front of her. He said, "Small girl, don't be afraid," and went away.

Her mother, a professor of criminal law, frequently entertained foreign academics at home. Elovainio, her brother and sister used to serve at the table and were exposed to numerous languages and cultures.

"I was very interested in pushing good news about cancer, the improvements in treatment and reduction in side effects. I was criticised for being too positive, but I was trying to counterbalance the bleak news."

The family moved to Helsinki when she was seven years old, and she has lived there ever since. Once qualified as a doctor, she practised only a few years before being offered the Health Promotion job at the Cancer Society. At first she missed seeing patients, and was unsure whether she would stay, but

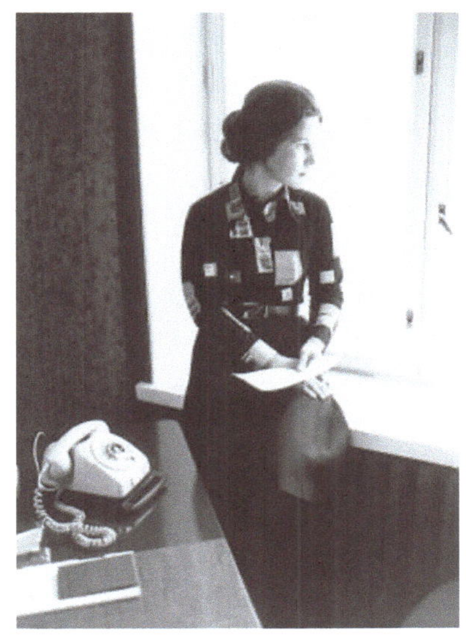

1974. Looking uncertain in the early days of a career at the Cancer Society of Finland

she became increasingly committed to her role. "It turned out to be so important and interesting. You can have some effect on the total population here. And when I started, in the 1970s, I was very interested in pushing good news about cancer, which had such a poor image. We systematically started to inform people of improving results with more effective and less toxic treatments. I was sometimes criticised for giving too positive a picture, but I was trying to counterbalance the bleak news that was everywhere."

On holiday in Capri. Dr. Elovainio (centre), with her mother (left)

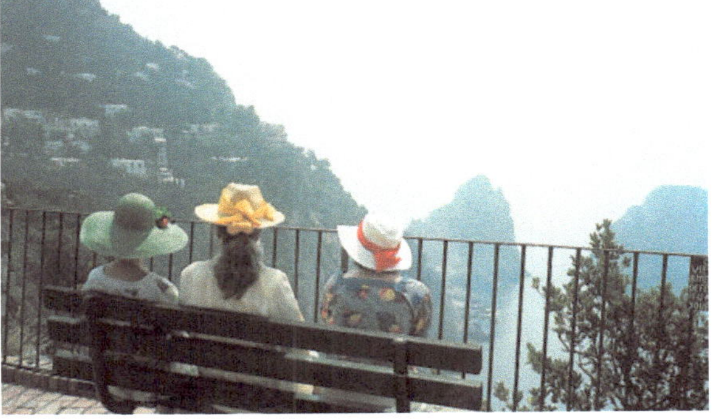

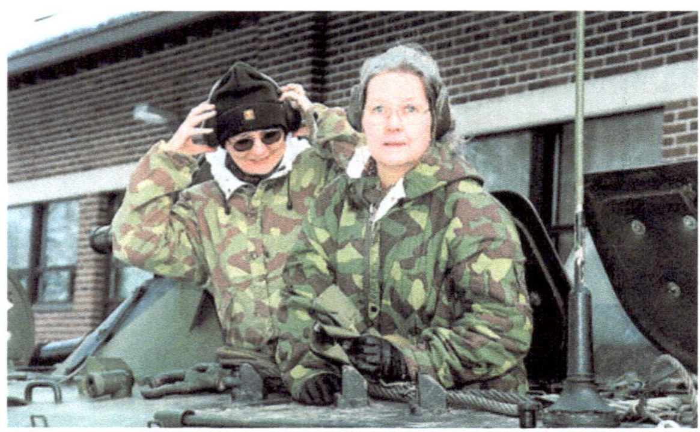

1996. Finnish top executives were invited by the Government to take part in an 8 week course on plans for a national emergency

Soon afterwards, the main Act on tobacco control came into force. She took a sabbatical and went to work for the Government, interpreting the Act and helping put it into practice. She had initially thought she might stay, but in the end was relieved to come back to the friendly and non-partisan atmosphere at the Cancer Society.

Since then, she has worked steadily and devotedly towards the promotion of health in Finland. "It's been a fantastically interesting career," she says. She has enjoyed working with the Cancer Society Board, top professionals, directors of banks and insurance companies, and professors. They are all unpaid, but bring in modern ways of thinking to keep the Society up to date. As Secretary General, she has been called upon, among other things, to undergo comprehensive security training for several weeks, so that she, along with other top professionals and chiefs of industry, can keep abreast of the plans for a national emergency. So she even used a gun once. "Fortunately, there was an ambulance standing by," she said.

Only a few weeks after first taking her job, she was asked by the military how many cigarettes they should set aside for emergency meetings in a bunker in a time of crisis. "How ironic that they should ask me! But you know, it was a good question, because somebody addicted to nicotine could not function in an emergency without tobacco," she says.

She made the same mistakes as everyone else in early campaigns, she says, but one of her favourites was based on the slogan, "If someone asks for a cigarette, offer a kiss instead." It was taken up and used abroad, but the sociologist in her refuses to take the credit for any effect it may have had. "There are always so many things going on. You never know, even afterwards, whether or not you have made a difference."

Her slogan, "If someone asks for a cigarette, offer a kiss instead" was even used abroad, but she refuses to take the credit for any effect. "You never know whether or not you have made a difference."

And yet, one of her greatest pleasures now is sitting in the audience of a cancer meeting and hearing a speaker referring to successes in Finland. "It makes me really happy," she says. Others are in no doubt about the effect she has had. She has won national and international medals and is a Knight of the Order of the Lion of Finland.

One of her awards came with a substantial amount of money. Elovainio does not have her own children, and used this money to enable her niece to have the treatment that allowed her to give birth to a son, now two years old. "I'm an honorary

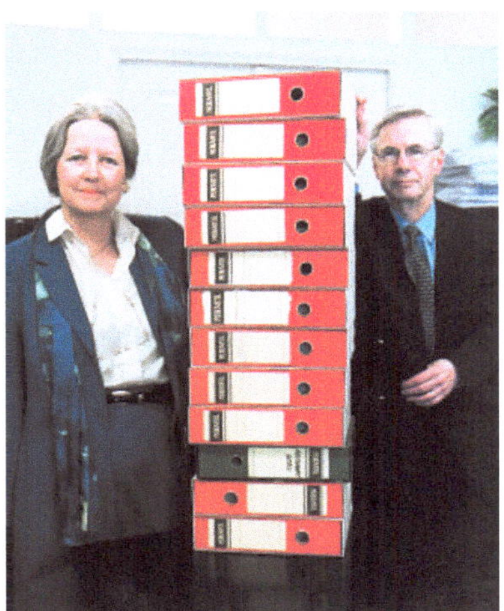

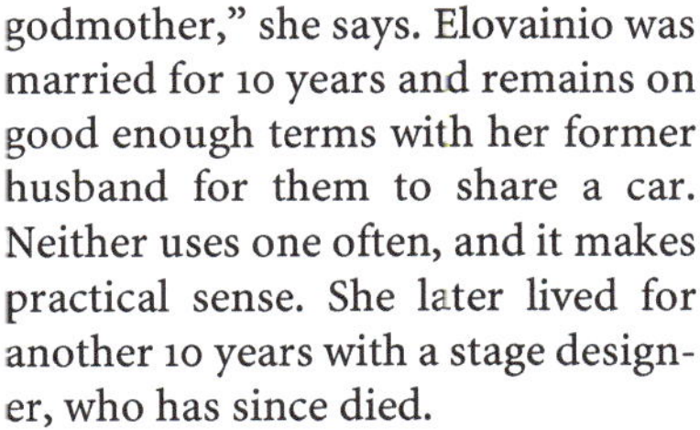

One year's applications for research funding! With Prof. Carl-Gustaf Standertskjöld Nordenstam, Chairman of the Finnish Cancer Foundation

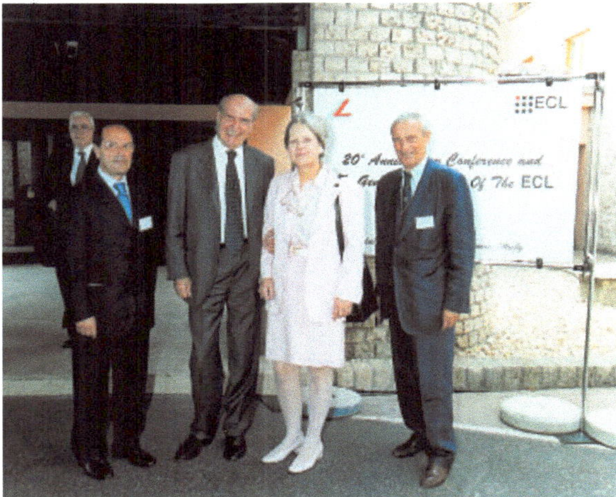

2000. In Rome with Dr. Francesco Schittulli (Italian Cancer League), Prof. Umberto Veronesi, Prof. Faosto Badellino (from left)

godmother," she says. Elovainio was married for 10 years and remains on good enough terms with her former husband for them to share a car. Neither uses one often, and it makes practical sense. She later lived for another 10 years with a stage designer, who has since died.

She enjoys her life in Helsinki, where she can walk to work and most of her meetings. She likes classical music and opera and collects pieces of art: paintings and sculpture depicting grand pianos. She has had an apartment in the French Riviera for years, and plans to spend more time there from next year, when she retires.

Her last big project is the organisation of the 12th World Conference on Tobacco or Health: Global Action for a Tobacco-Free Future. It is to be held in Helsinki in August 2003, and she wants it to be special. She is determinedly raising funds to pay the fares of the people who most need to be there: those from the developing world and Eastern Europe, currently so vulnerable to tobacco industry marketing.

After that, she says that she will retire from her job, and, once her term at the International Union Against Cancer comes to an end, from her role in cancer prevention. She will take a well-earned break and move into a new stage of life. It's hard to imagine one with so much energy, who has been so involved, simply departing, but she insists: "To my mind, if you're old and a bit out of things, you should not try to influence things. Cancer is so difficult, so complicated, it is impossible to be effective when you are not completely immersed in it."

Roche Oncology:

Leading the Way to Targeting Cancer with Care

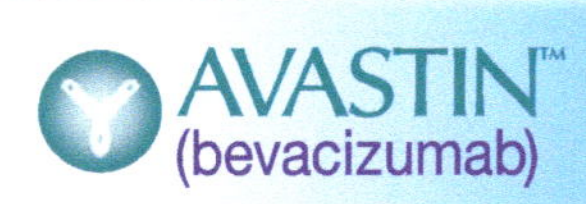

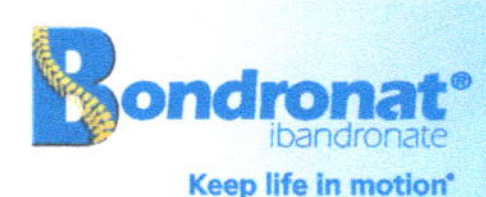

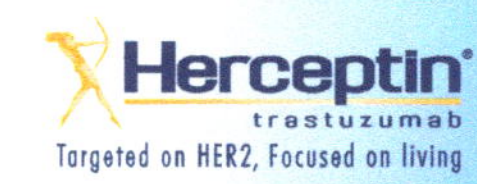

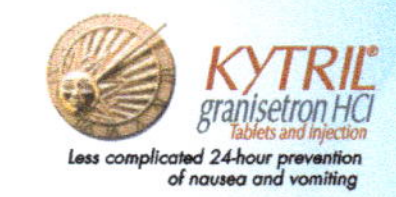

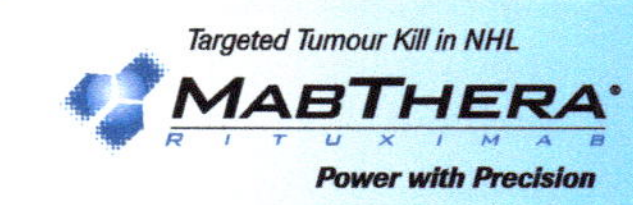

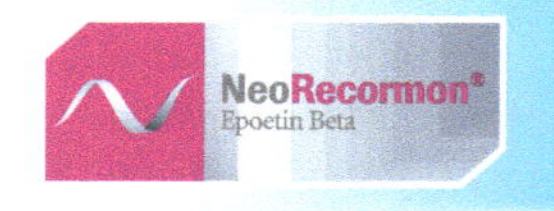

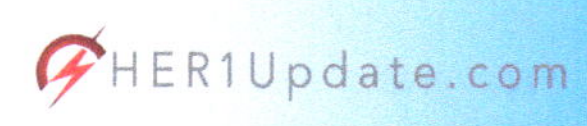

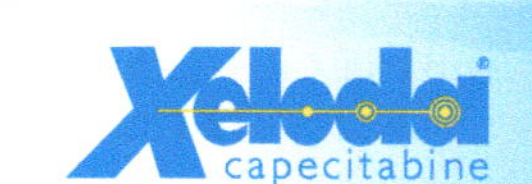

Franco Cavalli: Rebel with (Several) Rauses

Helen Saul

Under Fire, the 1983 film starring Nick Nolte, may have received lukewarm reviews by the critics, but, unbeknown to its creators, it is continuing to change the outlook for cancer patients throughout Central America. One audience in Europe contained Dr Franco Cavalli, oncologist and Swiss politician, and his date, oncology nurse Yvonne Willems. The film, set during the Nicaraguan civil war, started a chain reaction through their, and others', lives.

It made such an impression on Willems that she decided to go and see the country. Cavalli visited her there and went on to set up a non-governmental organisation (NGO) devoted to healthcare projects in Central America such as a new oncology department at a paediatric hospital in Managua and a radiotherapy centre in the same city. It was a logical, if dramatic, extension to his political and medical interests. And to his personal life. He and Willems not only married, but later adopted two young Nicaraguan boys. Quite a result.

Cavalli is an internationally renowned lymphoma specialist, and Director of the Oncology Institute of Southern Switzerland (OSSI). He is also a Member of Parliament, and has just stepped down as head of the Socialist Group at the Swiss Parliament because his responsibilities at OSSI are hitting a new high. The Institute has new premises, which are due to be opened in September 2002 by the Swiss Minister of Health. This is a milestone in the development of cancer services in the Italian-speaking part of Switzerland, and a source of personal satisfaction for Cavalli. He set up the services from scratch, almost 25 years ago.

In the meantime, he has also been a key player in the European Society for Medical Oncology (ESMO). He was one of a group who strove to take what was once essentially a French organisation, and make it European. He has been treasurer, executive committee member, and, for 10 years, founder and editor-in-chief of its journal, the Annals of Oncology. "When I launched it they were saying, 'In two years it will be dead;

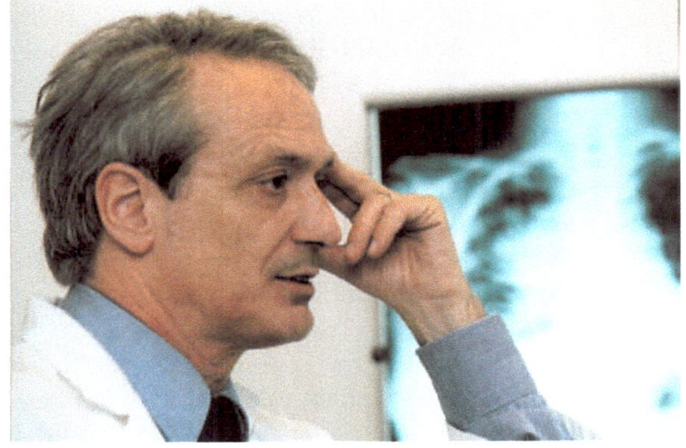

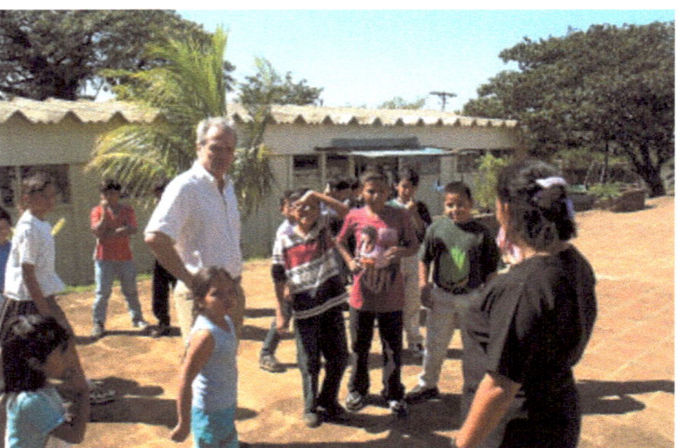

With the pupils of the school project "Barrilete de Colores", Managua, Nicaragua

it is impossible to do something like that in Europe'. Now Annals of Oncology is not only, from the clinical point of view, the best oncological journal, but it is approaching the level of American publications." And it's time for Cavalli to move on. He thrives on the impossible, is bored by the routine.

Yet, against these achievements, there is a certain modesty. He agrees to see me in extraordinary circumstances, only a few hours after he has had an emergency coronary angioplasty. I had already travelled to Switzerland, as arranged, in order to meet him at the Swiss Parliament in Bern. Instead of cancelling the meeting, he suggests we meet at the University hospital, where he is by now a patient. When I arrive, he looks well and relaxed and insists only that he has far longer than he would normally have to chat. He has had to cancel the speech he was due to give to Parliament that afternoon.

Cavalli's story is rooted in the Italian-speaking part of Switzerland, south of the Alps, a region of 500,000 people and home to his family for centuries. He was born and brought up in the village where his family have lived since his fore-

father, a powerful man in the Medici in Tuscany, lost a political battle and fled to the Alps. Even now, more than half of the village are called either Medici or Cavalli.

Politics is in the blood, and was frequently debated around the kitchen table.

He comes from a long line of political activists. His grandfather was a founder of the social democratic party in Italian-speaking Switzerland, and spent the Second World War helping freedom fighters from Italy to hide in Switzerland and then go back and fight. Politics is in the blood, and was frequently debated around the kitchen table.

It became more personal while he was still in his teens. The local Catholic school was free of charge for the village boys, but expensive for everyone else. "It was a period of social frustration for me, because all of the other pupils were the sons of rich families. If they went skiing, I had to say I didn't like it, because I didn't have any skis. But worse was the problem of how I could finance my studies at University. There were fellowships from the State, but only for outstanding pupils. The school's exam was set by an external committee who disapproved of private education, so they made it tough. It was terribly stressful for me because I not only had to pass, but I had to get a high average. I felt it was so unfair when my classmates could go out swimming when I had to study to get such high marks."

His dream was to become a journalist, having set up a local newspaper with his father when he was 14. His father wrote the local news and he wrote the international news, but the paper folded. Later, convinced that his son would starve as a journalist, Cavalli senior opposed this

He chose medicine finally, more by default than through conviction.

career choice. Cavalli himself discounted law as being full of lawyers carrying out dirty business, and engineering because of the unattractive mathematics. He chose medicine finally, more by default than through conviction.

He involved himself in the burgeoning student political movement, becoming vice-president of the Swiss Student Association. "All young people were interested in politics, because we still lived in an authoritarian system. I became politically active, following the political tradition of my family, which was left wing. I was perhaps a bit more left wing than they had been."

All the way through, his career has woven together politics and medicine. "I have two souls in one body," he says.

He qualified in 1968, and entered psychiatry. He had contacts with the anti-psychiatry movement, which was questioning the psychiatric methods of the time and aiming to open up clinics and wards. "But we didn't succeed, and the group fell apart like all the others after 1968."

The professor of medical oncology at Bern, who was also involved in politics, sparked Cavalli's interest in cancer, and he switched after two years to internal medicine, and later, to oncology. The decision was partly pragmatic. He wanted to be able to bring up his children in the Italian-

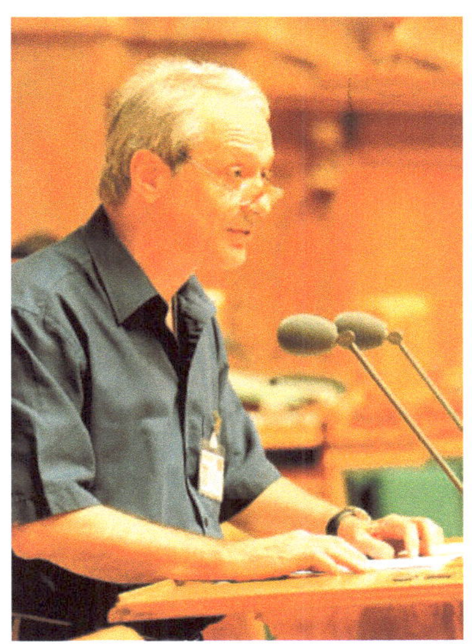

Speaking in Parliament

speaking part of Switzerland: with his first wife, he has four of his own children, one of whom died in an accident 10 years ago, and a further two children, adopted from Columbia. However, Cavalli had become known as a far-left agitator in the region, and his previous political campaigns limited his career choice. A direct attack on the chief of surgery in Lugano for earning huge amounts by employing other people rather than carrying out any work himself did not make him any friends in that quarter.

"In oncology, there was nothing, there was nobody else."

"Everyone from the roadsweeper to the most important doctor was selected by political considerations. If I had been a gynaecologist, and there were others with the same qualifications, I would have had problems. But in oncology, there was nothing, there was nobody else."

In 1978, he moved back to Bellinzona to set up a division of oncology at the Ospedale San Giovanni. The next year, along with Dr Bonnadonna from Milan, he organised a conference in Lugano on treatment questions in testicular lymphoma for the International Union Against Cancer (UICC). Together, they proposed the "watch and see" policy for seminal lymphomas, and the meeting was a success. It has been held every third year since then, and is a fixture on the calendars of all those dealing with lymphoma.

Organising the ensuing conference put Cavalli in touch with leaders in the field, and propelled his own career in lymphoma. At the same time, he was starting to build up a cancer service. There was so much infighting within the region that patients were often referred to Geneva or Zurich, outside of the region altogether, rather than to local colleagues. "Everyone with cancer had to go north, to French- or German-speaking regions, which for many was very stressful, as not all are fluent in these languages. There are many blue-collar workers here, and it also put a financial strain on their families. I have always been in favour of patients staying near home and close to their primary physician,

and wanted to create something so that everyone can be treated for cancer here."

In less than 25 years, a full and modern cancer ervice has emerged.

In 1978, he started, with half a nurse and half a secretary, to make this happen. In less than 25 years, a full and modern cancer service has emerged, as a combination of centralised and decentralised care, based at the OSSI and four main hospitals: in Bellinzona, the political capital, Locarno and Lugano. The new building in Bellinzona will bring most of the activities together, provide patients with everything from prevention to palliative care and continue as a leading centre in research in the specialist fields of breast cancer, lymphoma, and new drugs. It will have 35 beds for radiotherapy and medical oncology, arranged over two floors, with patients divided according to how sick they are, rather than whether they are to receive radiotherapy or chemotherapy.

OSSI's research achievements are remarkable for an institute in such a small region, and have been made possible by international collaboration. First in lymphoma, Cavalli's own speciality. The Lugano conference is routinely attended by leaders from around the globe. Cavalli's reputation means patients are referred to him from outside the region, and he therefore sees far more than would occur among such a small population. He established the International Extranodal Lymphoma Study Group (IELSG) five years ago, to study the 40% of lympho-

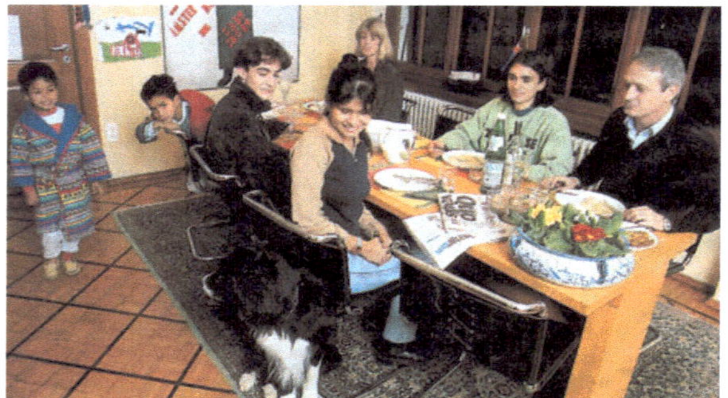

Franco and Yvonne with five of their seven children (José, Stefano, Samuele, Laura and Daniele)

mas that arise in tissues other than the lymph nodes, such as the brain, stomach, liver or lung. The organ of origin is of paramount importance in predicting outcome, in that, for example, lymphomas of the salivary glands are cured in 80% of cases, whereas testicular or central nervous system lymphomas are cured in only 10–15%. No institution would have enough cases of bone lymphomas, say, to study the disease alone, so cooperative groups are essential. The IELSG includes about 40 institutions from Europe, Asia and the Americas, and has almost 500 cases of testicular lymphomas. "In the literature before us, you would see series of 45 or 50 patients," he says.

Breast cancer research at OSSI is led by Dr Aron Goldhirsch, who has worked with Cavalli for 20 years and is another international heavyweight. He heads the International Breast Cancer Study Group, which, after an American group, is the second most important breast cancer group worldwide. Goldhirsch spends half his time at OSSI and the rest at the European Institute of Oncology in Milan.

New drugs research is headed by Cavalli, assisted by Dr Christianna Sessa, who again spends half her time at OSSI and half at the Tumour Institute in Milan. Sessa, who is responsible for phase I trials and clinical pharmacology, and conducts trials based between the two centres, often finds she is able to start programmes at OSSI six months to a year before she can get through the Italian bureaucracy to get going in Milan.

Allied with OSSI is the Institute for Biomedical Research, set up in response to Roche's closure of its

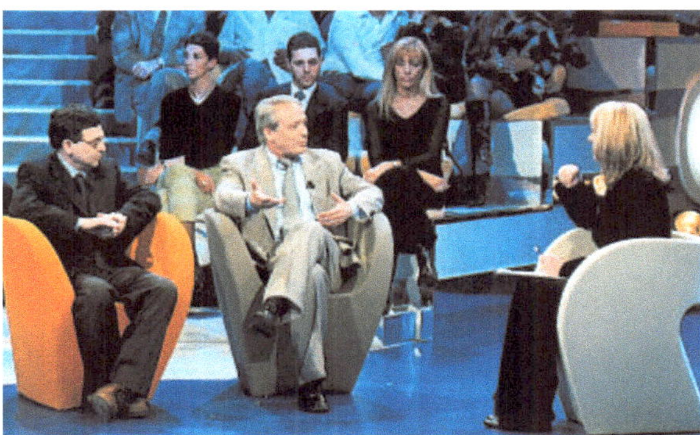

2002. Appearing with Dr Catapano, head of research labs in Lugano, on a Swiss TV talk show, to raise money for cancer research

Basle Institute of Immunology. It is headed by Dr Lanzavechia, a renowned specialist in dendritic cells, and employs many of his former colleagues from the Basle Institute. The current plan is to move OSSI's research laboratories into this institute, to bring together basic and translational research. "It will be interesting from a synergistic point of view," Cavalli says.

> **"Many physicians have been spoilt, they have earned too much, and lost the confidence of their patients who think they are only interested in money."**

But Cavalli is rushing on. Yes, they have a new building, and he wants to consolidate its situation as the "first really comprehensive cancer centre in Switzerland." But more than that, he wants it to be at least as good as the American centres, "maybe better in some aspects," and to be a role model for other centres in Europe. In the way it is financed, for example. Here the medic and politician merge. "The problem of increasing costs in healthcare and the reforms which are needed represent political issue number one in Switzerland. Many physicians have been spoilt,

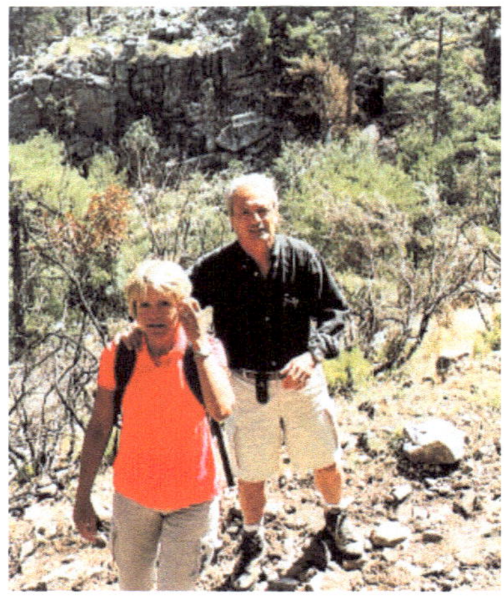

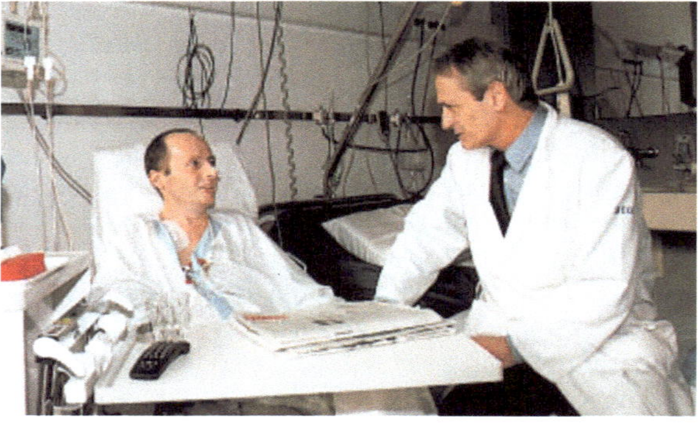

At work in the
hospital

a higher salary. But it is quite usual for patients to have extra insurance, and in the new centre this will be for the benefit of the hospital, not the individual doctors' wallets.

Politics are never far from the surface in talking to Cavalli. He was unable to be politically active when first setting up the cancer services, and he found that difficult. "I had to work 24 hours a day to build up the services, and it was simply impossible for me to also be involved in politics. I suffered because of that. I mean, I even suffer if I'm on holiday and cannot get hold of the New York Times. I need to know what's going on."

After the enforced break during the first years back in southern Switzerland, Cavalli returned to politics in 1985, this time as member of the regional parliament in Canton Ticino. It was a position he held for 10 years. His high profile as a cancer doctor has given him a popularity in the region that has exempted him from needing to carry out election campaigns. "Every family here has at least one relative treated by me or my co-workers," he says.

"It was a short hop back to Bern in October 1995, when he was elected to the Swiss Parliament, and since then he has divided his time fairly equally between oncology and politics. His views have remained fairly constant, he says.

they have earned too much, and lost the confidence of their patients who think they are only interested in money." This will not be possible in the new centre. In Switzerland, everyone has to take out a basic health insurance package, but complementary insurance packages are needed for extra frills such as a single room, choice of surgeon, alternative treatments and some kinds of plastic surgery. Cavalli himself does not take private patients – "For cancer patients, the idea of having to differentiate between patients according to money would be very much against my principles" – and to take account of this, the government awards him

budgets in healthcare, provided they are used correctly and not in the interests of the establishment. But basically my position has not changed a lot.

"The Socialist party in Switzerland represents one-quarter of those who vote – 25%. And we have a proportional system here, which means we take 25% of the seats in parliament. Ours is one of four big parties, in general the biggest one, and usually the parties build a coalition to form a government. Most of the time, even if we are in the government, we vote against it, and that is absolutely acceptable. If we disagree with a law that has been passed and can gather enough support, we can ask for a referendum, and get the people to vote. So citizens participate here rather more than in most European countries. We have made use of the referendum on issues such as limitation on the numbers of foreign refugees and liberalisation of the energy market, both of which we opposed. We are obliged to keep closely in contact with the public because of this system, and in fact the Swiss Socialist Party is somewhat further to the left than most others in Europe, which is strange."

The developing world has long been a focus of Cavalli's interest. "Nations in the southern part of the world cannot become more independent from the north and develop economically, because they are largely exploited. Their fight to do so has to be an important part not only of the activity, but of the vision of someone who is left-wing."

During the Algerian and Vietnam wars, he was involved in "liberation committees", and saw devel-

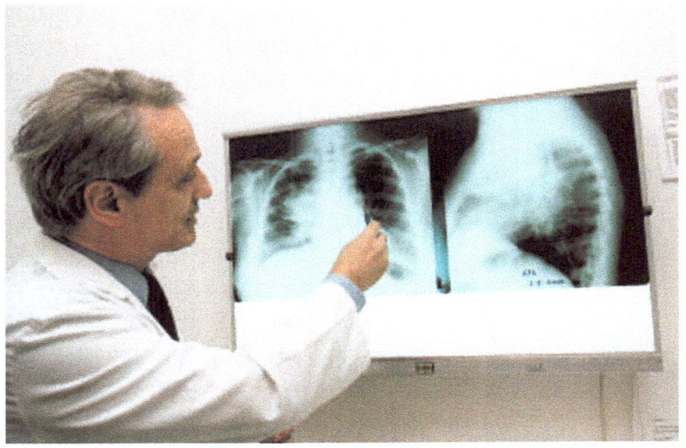

opment as a purely political issue. But as he progressed in his medical career, he became increasingly concerned about healthcare issues. This belief has translated into a deep involvement with projects in Central America, such as a plant for the production of cytotoxic drugs in Havana, Cuba.

Ventures require long-term commitment, and the key, he says, is heavy initial investment, which tapers off as the project becomes independent.

So a new hospital requires a building, training for physicians, nurses, lab technicians and so on, equipment and drugs, plus a guesthouse for family members to make it possible for people to come. But alongside that, local people have to be involved in fundraising so that it can continue into the future.

Technology needs to be kept as simple as possible. "Avoid everything which is not absolutely essential," says Cavalli. "Too many Americans go in and say: 'We know how it has to be done, you have to have a drug which costs $500, go and buy it!' This helps nobody. We try to adapt our technology to their conditions as far as possible, and you don't have to spend billions. You can use it in a much less expensive way.

"When we started our project in paediatric leukaemia, all the children died. In Europe we have a cure rate of perhaps 80% and now, in Managua, it is 50%.

Some of those who are not cured probably cannot be cured because they are so weak, or are living in such poor conditions that even by taking care of the leukaemia they would die of a strange infection. To achieve the same results as here, you would need to have the same conditions – the water should be as clear and so on – and that's impossible for us. But if you can cure 50% of these children, it is important, and it can only be achieved through an effort that in the end will also profit a lot of other people in the hospital."

Cavalli's concerns about developing countries are so much a part of his world view that, with or without the prompt of that Hollywood film, his very own blend of medical and political, social and personal, vision and pragmatism would have been put to good use somewhere. But it does make you wonder what would have happened in Managua if he and Willems had decided that evening to go to a restaurant rather than the cinema.

Françoise Meunier: Chameleon Chief

Helen Saul

Françoise Meunier, Director General of the European Organisation
for Research and Treatment of Cancer (EORTC), has two things on her mind
when we meet. One is her current priority to ensure that the European
Directive on clinical trials is implemented in such a way that it guarantees
the future of collaborative research. The other is the delivery
of a six-metre-high Ginkgo Biloba tree – an extraordinary present
to her husband for their 15th wedding anniversary.

Meunier is a multifaceted personality. She is a self-confessed "tough cookie", fierce in her determination to advance the cause of cancer research and treatment. At the same time, she exudes an unexpected playfulness and eccentricity. Her husband and daughter describe her variously as serene, sensitive, loyal, dominant and hedonistic.

**She is like a hermit crab,
her daughter says, changing
shells to suit the occasion.**

For work, she dons an indestructible shell, radiating enthusiasm and dynamism. At home she is still commanding, and ready to move mountains for those she loves, but the shell is more fragile. Her husband agrees. "She's a chameleon!" he says.

Her working life certainly demands a degree of robustness. As Director General, she has a pivotal role in pan-European cancer research. She co-ordinates all EORTC's activities and ensures they fit into the strategies defined by the Board, General Assembly and various committees. She co-ordinates the organisation of conferences, and is a fundraiser and a spokeswoman for EORTC and for cancer in general. She is, she says, a medical manager.

Yet, until 1991, she was an ambitious young professor, head of Infectious Diseases at the renowned Jules Bordet Institute in Brussels. She changed direction on 3 January 1991,

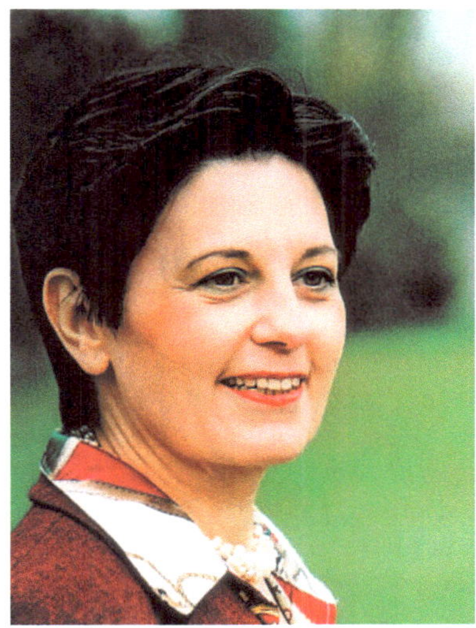

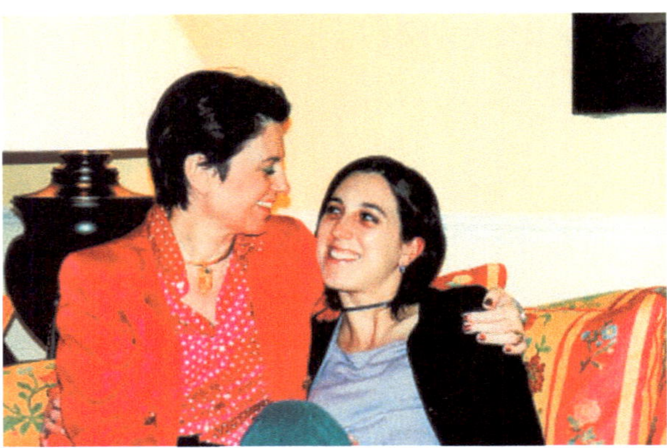

With daughter
Caroline

after a visit to the Institute's former director, Henri Tagnon, to wish him a Happy New Year. It turned out to be an important social call. He told her that the EORTC Data Center was looking for a director, and suggested she apply.

Meunier's career at Jules Bordet – where EORTC was established and housed until 1990 – meant she was familiar with the organisation and what it stood for, and it seemed a golden opportunity. "The whole spirit of Bordet was to randomise patients, and participate in international groups and activities. It was an ideal setting, a goal to reach, it meant participating in the international scene. I knew the value and potential of EORTC. Being an idealist, I fit into it very well. I was raised in the spirit of improving, scientific rigour, intellectual honesty and an enquiring, discerning mind."

It meant leaving a high-flying academic career, but Meunier had made her mind up in a week. "The decision was made quickly, because I am not one to hesitate. When I take a decision, I go for it, I look forward and I never have any regrets. It's my way. I take whatever consequences there are."

Her arrival at EORTC was a baptism of fire.

This is just as well, because her arrival at EORTC was a baptism of fire. The organisation was in a financial crisis; new national and international laws governing clinical practice and trials were appearing, and the Data Center was suffering from a lack of medical input – Meunier herself was the only MD on the staff. She went to the Board and suggested a wholesale restructuring, including new units for quality of life, health economics, monitoring and regulatory affairs. They gave her their backing, with the proviso that she herself find the money to carry out the changes.

Just to make things harder, she set up the EORTC Fungal Infections Group as soon as she arrived. This was a natural follow-on from her academic work, and she chaired it until 1995. But she was building it from scratch at the same time as restructuring the Data Center.

It was a testing introduction, even for the steely side of Meunier. "I was asked at my interview whether I could fire people, and I understood from the beginning that there would be problems, but not to the extent I found. Some of the internal staff were like little queens over their departments, and I kept hearing 'On a toujours fait comme cela, Madame' – it is always done this way. It's a sentence I hate, because it means they want to continue in the same way. So I met some resistance and had to fire several staff; others left of their own accord.

"But my reward is that, 10 years later, everybody agrees that I was right, and now nobody either inside or outside of the EORTC could imagine a Data Center without medical doctors. The staff are happy, the groups have a better professional service."

Change was rapid. "We had no choice. It was that and survival, or die," says Meunier. Medical fellows started arriving within months, and Patrick Therasse and Denis Lacombe were among the first group. Now respectively Director of the Data Center and Assistant Director of Drug Development, she describes them as her right and left arm. "I was lucky because they are outstanding. They understood my philosophy and final objective and we agreed on the strategy. I did not rescue the EORTC alone."

She also says that she has been well supported by the Executive and the Presidents – professors with their own departments who work for the EORTC on a voluntary basis. Even so, she has had to be assertive. Hers is a direct approach, fuelled by a passion for the cause she supports, and she says it comes naturally. "I am not saying that I am very diplomatic. People know if I am happy, they know if I am unhappy.

> **"When I have to say something, I say it bluntly. I am rough and tough, and somehow I don't make a great effort to hide it because I am always doing it for the best."**

If something goes wrong, I am not happy and I have to say so. Everybody knows that I am the boss."

Meunier views it as a privilege to work for the EORTC. She admits that she is demanding on her staff; she is also demanding on herself. She

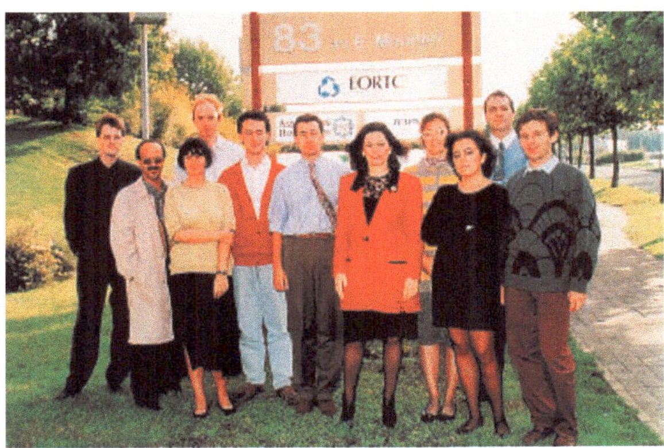

Meunier with her first group of fellows at EORTC in 1993

is dedicated and committed and expects the same of others. Staff phone her every morning, even when she's on holiday. If something is promised, she will pursue it until it arrives. Her persistence is apparent, in and outside of work: "I don't know anyone else who can get a plumber to come within an hour of a call!" says her husband.

Equally, when she receives requests from patients, she is careful to reply promptly. Queries about second opinions, clinical trials, appropriate treatment, or anything else, are dealt with within 24 hours. She enjoys this continuing link with patients.

The EORTC provides an infrastructure for independent academic research. It now encompasses expertise in regulatory affairs, ethics, tumour banks, translational research, health economics, quality of life and all aspects of research. Units are set up as the need arises and disbanded when redundant. It is a dynamic network.

A European directive, intended to improve the situation, has been passed by the European Parliament. However, Meunier says that national authorities have been given too

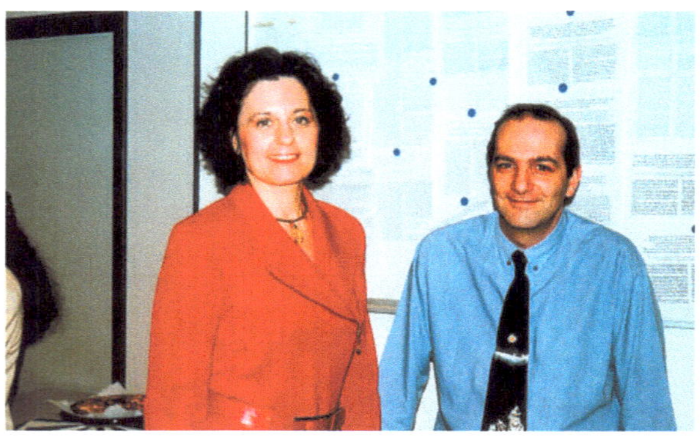

much leeway to introduce their own clauses. Nation states have to implement the Directive by May 2003 and apply it by May 2004. "We are now at a critical point where we have to make national authorities understand the challenge for European research. If each of them accumulates contradictory or extravagant requirements, or extra bureaucracy, it will slow down European research and advancement. At just the moment when the Sixth Framework is being launched by the Commission, aiming to integrate facilities, build networks and improve the European research area, it is really not the time to put obstacles in the way.

Meunier's current priority is the harmonisation of the laws relating to research across Europe.

"In Europe, we have the brains, we have the expertise, we have the know-how, the patients, the facilities, everything. But if you are trying to carry out translational research and it becomes a nightmare to move tissue samples across borders, research will suffer. If we want networking throughout Europe, we must remove unnecessary barriers."

A position paper from the European Forum on Good Clinical Practice (Brussels, September 2001, updated December 2002) estimates that costs of clinical trials could increase by 30% if procedures are not streamlined across Europe. Authorities, in effect, demand documentation they already have. They have the full dossier for all approved drugs, for example, but sponsors initiating a trial have to provide it again. Information has to be produced in a variety of languages, and in various formats, because there is no common form. "None of these extra demands increases the quality of science or patient protection. They add bureaucracy and administration without improving the science," she said. Another danger is that pan-European research becomes so slow and so complicated to set up that it is easier simply to conduct trials elsewhere, in the US or Japan.

"None of these extra demands increases the quality of science or patient protection. They add bureaucracy and administration without improving the science."

Meunier is optimistic – as she always is – that this will not happen, and she is co-ordinating various efforts to tackle the issue. She has become a public advocate, cares passionately about the subject and gets intensely frustrated when progress is not always smooth. "Sometimes you get the feeling that you have to go against the world to make things change. Things may seem obvious to you, but others do not necessarily perceive the same needs or challenges. It is frustrating when I am not convincing or effective enough, or when there are other reasons for not achieving goals like this more rapidly or effectively."

She seems so embroiled in the issue that it's hard to imagine how she'll move on once national laws are in place and she can do little more. But she rattles off a list of other pre-occupations, including EORTC's health economics conference in 2003 and revitalisation of exchange programmes with the US' National Cancer Institute (NCI).

Top of the list, though, is the issue of insurance for patients entering clinical trials.

Many ethical committees insist that patients are insured by a company based in their own country. This complicates pan-European trials and, in any case, contradicts a European Directive on the freedom to provide services. Meunier intends to raise awareness of the problem, as soon as she is finished with harmonisation. She is enthusiastic about all of her causes and says that the moment one issue is resolved another takes its place. Her mission is to maintain EORTC as the reference pan-European cancer research organisation, and she will take on any challenge to cancer research. Whatever it may be.

It is all so very different from the career in clinical medicine that Meunier envisaged, even as a child. Her father was a surgeon in a coun-

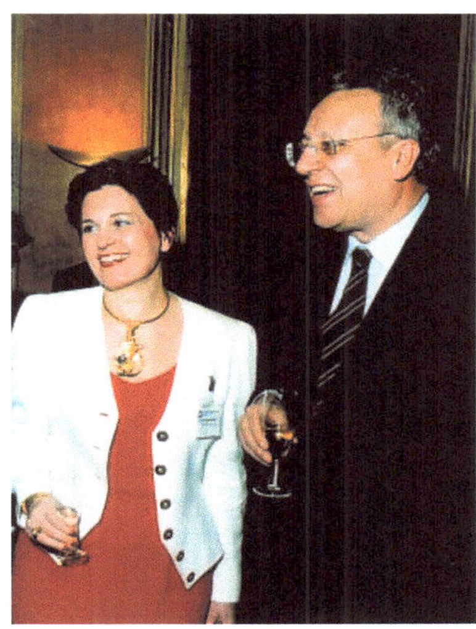

With Philippe Busquin, EU Commissioner for Research, EORTC's 40th anniversary, Brussels, March 2002

try town not far from Brussels, so she had some idea what it entailed. She was close to her father. They enjoyed each others' intellect and joie de vivre, and from him she learned her love of good food and wine. In fact, one of her greatest regrets is that he died shortly after she started at EORTC and before she could show him round. "He would have been so proud," she said. She is also still close to her brother, who is younger and was similarly influenced by their father. He went on to be a vet. Meunier says she might have enjoyed archeology or history, but neither were real possibilities. She was always going to be a doctor, and it was not a difficult decision.

She liked the way that the department was trying to improve treatments and was fascinated by its clinical trials.

As a student she worked in the infectious diseases department at Jules Bordet. She liked the way that the department was trying to im-

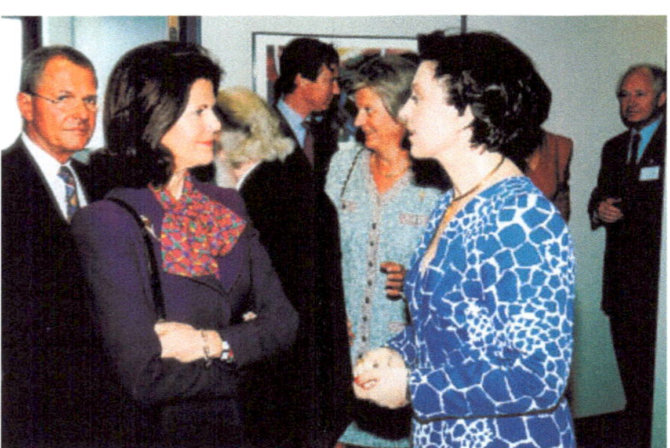

With Queen Sylvia of Sweden, Honorary President of the EORTC Foundation, who visited the headquarters in 1998

prove treatments and was fascinated by its clinical trials, an approach less evident in other hospitals where she trained. She worked with Prof. Jean Klastersky, then head of Infectious Diseases, and started in his department in 1972.

At the time, leukaemic patients were receiving intensive chemotherapy and then dying of bacterial infections, of gram-negative septicaemia. The EORTC Antimicrobial Therapy Group, set up in 1974, initiated major studies to try to develop new ways of using antibiotics to decrease the mortality of these patients. The group showed that antibiotics should be given as soon as patients developed fever, rather than waiting to identify the cause, because patients could die before the results came back from the lab. It was extremely difficult: "Patients were young and we lost them often, too often. It was hard, but we could see progress and that was rewarding. But by 1976, when we had started to make progress on gram-negative septicaemia, another challenge arrived, and it was fungal."

Patients were dying of deep-seated fungal infections. Meunier was summoned by Professor Tagnon

and told that she would have to go to the US to research and study for a PhD. There was little interest in fungal infections in Europe at the time.

She and her first husband were duly despatched to New York. Meunier had married young, when she was 20, and only three years into her medical training. She changed university at the same time, from the Catholic University of Leuven to the Free University of Brussels, where her husband, already a doctor, worked. Her contemporaries were convinced she would drop out of university, which is perhaps what drove her on. She graduated as top student, Maxima cum Laude, which was what first brought her to the attention of Professor Tagnon.

In New York, she studied fungal infections at Memorial Sloan Kettering, while her husband, a surgeon, went to Columbia University. They worked hard, loved Manhatten life, and stayed two years. Her managerial side was already active, she says, and, knowing that she was coming back to Brussels at the end of 1978, she decided to have a baby in between jobs. "My daughter was born in September, we came back at the end of November, I started work in January and never had maternity leave."

This, of course, meant finishing off her work at Memorial and her publication virtually as soon as she had given birth, and having only a few weeks to settle back into Brussels before starting a new job.

She wrote her thesis in the evenings once her daughter, Caroline, was in bed, but dismisses this as being the same for many clinicians.

She never considered looking for a part-time job, she always knew she wanted to be active in her career and was obviously prepared to put in the hours to make it happen.

Her first husband was another career academic and, partly as a result, the marriage faltered. With her normal matter-of-fact attitude, when she decided it was over, she did not dither or hesitate. "When I decided to end the marriage, I went in another direction and that was that." She and her husband remained close and shared the care of Caroline, who was five years old at the time of the split. Both were frequent travellers and it was complicated, but they compared diaries 6 months in advance, agreed on where Caroline would be, and managed a difficult situation amicably. Even if it often seemed that Caroline almost always had one parent out of the country.

Every aspect of her life seems to be carefully managed. But underneath the no-nonsense exterior lies a more complex character. According to her family, she can lose several nights' sleep because of a colleague's personal or professional problems. The colleague will never know anything about it. She also has an unusual awareness of the fragility of life, and of death. "When I leave home in the morning, I always wonder whether I am going to comeback.

I am very aware of the fact that at any moment I may drop dead, or my husband or daughter have an accident. I think about death often."

These thoughts may be a result of her earlier work with dying leukaemia patients, perhaps heightened by

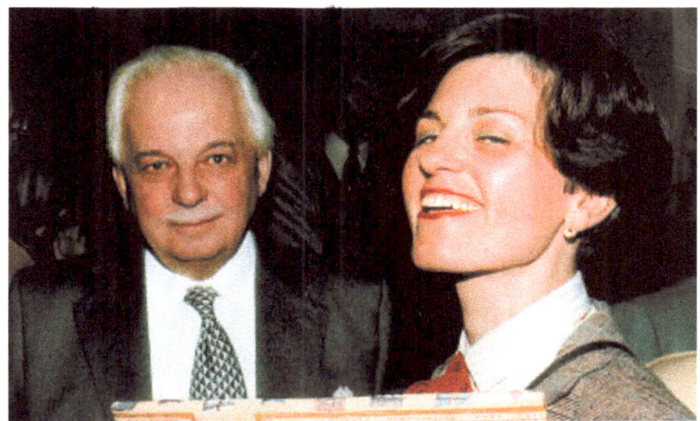

Meunier with her father, at her PhD graduation, 1985

the knowledge that her second husband, Jean-Marie, was treated for cancer 20 years ago. Whatever the origin, her response is remarkable. She and Jean-Marie have already had their grave built, in the village where he lives outside of Brussels. Both have their signatures embodied in stone. He is an eminent notary, and both have signed so many documents in their lives they decided to have signatures rather than an elaborate decoration. The stone has her birthdate with a space for the date of death, and a simple description, that she was Director General of the EORTC and mother of Caroline Carpentier. "I absolutely must have that on my gravestone," she says.

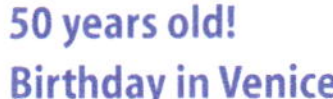

50 years old! Birthday in Venice

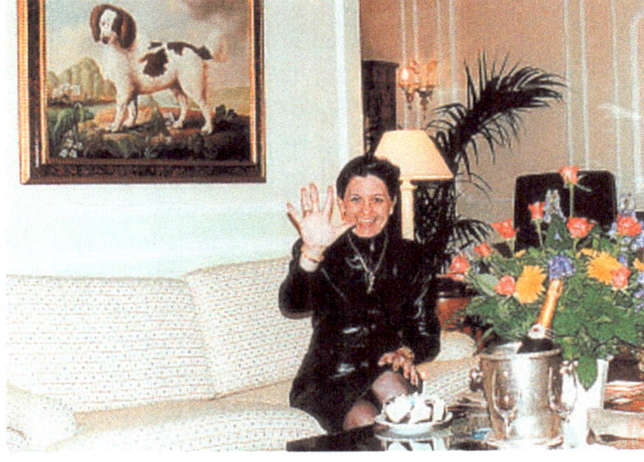

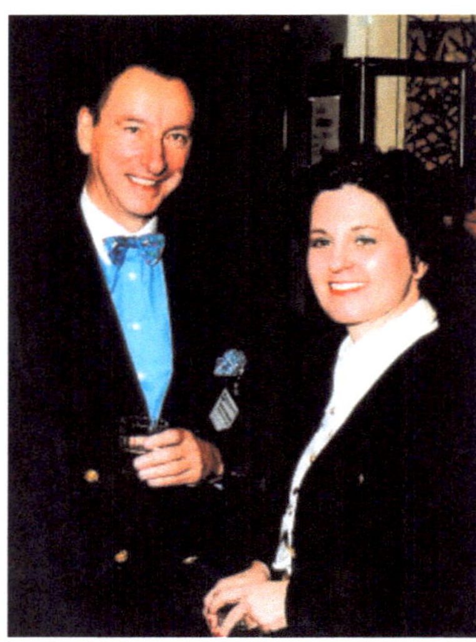

With her husband at EORTC's 40th anniversary celebration

Meunier's careful planning for the future covers not only death but deterioration. A few years ago, she bought the house next door to her own and completely renovated it so that she will be able to live there if she ever becomes handicapped or disabled. It is a large and beautiful home, with room for a live-in nurse and all the facilities she would need, however incapacitated. This seems to take organisation to bizarre lengths, but Meunier says that many people are afraid of speaking or thinking about death.

Her approach, she says, is one of taming death by making straightforward plans and dealing with it.

Part of the incentive is that Jean-Marie is 15 years her elder, and she is aware that he could "disappear" before her. Another is that they do not want either her daughter or his children and grandchildren – he has 11 – to have to make all the arrangements in the event of one of their deaths. But thoughts of death appear to be deep-rooted and complex, and it is tempting to wonder whether the Ginkgo Biloba, which she describes as highly symbolic, the first to grow up after the destruction in Hiroshima, may represent a desire to defy death. "It's the tree of eternity," she says.

Maybe. But in any case it's an incredible present, perhaps simply an extravagant gesture. Certainly, all talk of ageing and decline contrast sharply with the more obvious impression of a woman at the height of her powers professionally, while brimming over with affection for her husband and daughter. Her second marriage has been "exemplary", she says. By the time she met Jean-Marie, she had grown up and was more like the person she is today. It was also a second marriage for him, and he knew what he wanted and expected from the relationship. They share the same rules, she says, the same basic philosophy and the same approach to life. "We have never had a cross word in 15 years", she says.

Meunier is also immensely proud of her daughter, now 24 and a recently qualified lawyer. She left home only a few months ago, but still lives near enough to pop round to borrow olive oil or a whisk at 10 o'clock at night. Meunier dispenses recipes down the phone, they go shopping together, and for years they took an annual holiday, just the two of them. They visited capital cities throughout Europe and the rest of the world.

Her daughter, she says, was in a difficult position, with two academics for parents and then Jean-Marie, "somebody who takes up a lot of room," another achiever. But Caroline has become her own person, with a strong sense of social responsibility. As a student, she helped build a school in Peru; now she values her legal work with people who cannot afford to pay as highly as the big cases on intellectual property. Meunier cherishes the relationship.

She also has a good life with Jean-Marie. During the week she lives mainly in her house in the City; he commutes from there a few days a week. They make full use of the museums, galleries, bookshops and restaurants. She loves every kind of music, pop to classical. At the weekend, they go out to his house in the country. One of her greatest pleasures is to spend a whole Sunday picking fruit and vegetables in the garden.

She enjoys reading, some history but mostly biographies. She's always fascinated by how the subjects face major challenges and come through them; on holiday, she can get through three biographies in a week.

She enjoys reading biographies. She's always fascinated by how the subjects face major challenges and come through them.

She has fresh flowers delivered to her office every week (and then is billed for them at home). She has a pool at home and swims often, though not every day. Her personal trainer comes round every week puts

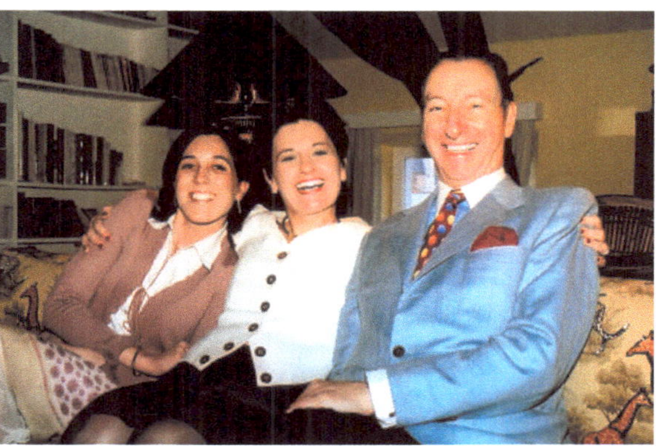

A relaxing family weekend at home

her through her paces, after which she sleeps like a baby. Caroline says she is "in full bloom, surfing on a wave and smiling at life." Jean-Marie says that he has seen no faults in her at all, except that when she washes her hair under the shower she gets water all over the bathroom. Including on the ceiling.

And this, after 15 years of marriage. At the dinner they held to celebrate the anniversary, Caroline arrived with a beautiful tree, a symbolic, slow-growing, long-living plant. Manageable, though, as a Bonzai. The Ginkgo Biloba, weighing in at six tonnes, was a bit more trouble. It took a huge truck, a revolving crane and three metres of earth to get it into the ground, but the operation was a success. Which is not surprising, because when Meunier has set her heart on something, you can be sure that mere details won't stop her.

Jean-Pierre Armand: Sifting Sand

HELEN SAUL

It's a long time since French oncologist Jean-Pierre Armand was working on an archeological dig in Greece (as a pre-clinical medical student, he found the summer breaks the most interesting part). Combing through dust and dirt, looking for hidden clues to tell an ancient story. In his student days, almost before the ink on his exam papers was dry, he would be off, leaving Toulouse to hitchhike his way through southern Europe and the Middle East. On occasion he would spend a month with archeologists in Dellos, Greece, offering his services in return for the pleasure of understanding more about the work.

Nowadays, he works from a modest office, every surface crammed with papers, at the Institut Gustave-Roussy in Villejuif, just outside Paris. As a working environment, it could hardly be more different from the open skies of the Greek archeological site. But he describes his work in phase I trials in similar terms. He loves the independence he has to do the best he possibly can for patients for whom there is no standard treatment. It gives him freedom from the guidelines and protocols so rife throughout oncology. An explorer at heart, he is driven by the search for useful compounds among many potential but ultimately flawed candidates. In spirit at least, Armand is still sifting sand.

He has been head of the Phase I Unit at the Institut Gustave-Roussy since 1984, but he remains a general oncologist, which is more difficult than it used to be, and his enthusiasm shows no sign of waning. His patients are in a bad way and may have tumours for which existing treatments are unsatisfactory, such as a brain or head and neck tumour, or tumours that have relapsed or failed to respond to a standard treatment. Results are often poor, but Armand maintains, "It's happening work, especially at present when we have a lot of fantastic drugs arriving. Patients don't have a reference treatment, and it is not clear what you should do, so you have more

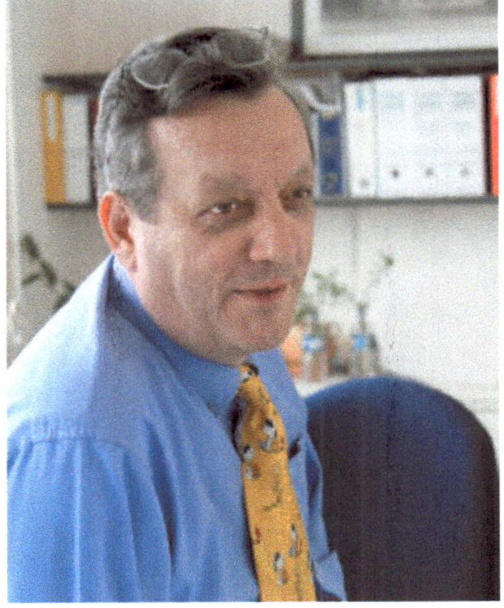

freedom to offer the benefit of your years of clinical experience.

"We are the first to approach new drugs, and it is a privilege, difficult but interesting."

Sometimes our success rates are not fantastic, but you always feel you can make a difference."

Armand's day to day work is based at the Institut Gustave-Roussy, but his influence spans France and Europe. For a start, he is President of the Societé Française du Cancer (SFC), which publishes the Bulletin du cancer and advises the authorities. It's an auspicious time, because President Jacques Chirac is backing a five-year campaign against cancer. It will offer both money and political will, and will encompass prevention, tobacco control, and early detection. All cancer structures in France are to be restructured around cancer centres in order to improve patients' access to treatment and drugs. And there will be a whole-hearted effort to promote translational research, an area close to his heart. Armand: "In France we are strong basic research-ers and very good clinicians, but in between the links are not good. We need some input in improving this connection." Armand has until April to come up with original proposals to offer the campaign the maximum chance of success.

Next, he is Chairman of the Groupe de Travail sur les Médicaments Anticancéreux (GTMAC), which advises the French Minister of Health on the registration of drugs. Armand lists his part in early registration of three key drugs – taxotere, irinotecan and oxaliplatin – as one of the highlights of his career. These drugs were licensed in France before other European countries – and seven years before the US in the case of oxaliplatin. Armand argued for this on the basis of clinical experience and a strong feeling that they would be useful. But it was before firm evidence existed on paper. "It was not clear that this would be a success, and we had to take a risk to offer the drug to patients more quickly than other countries in the world. For my patients, it was fantastic."

This pushy stance is, Armand says, typical of the French approach. "The British are more conservative and wait longer to offer new drugs to patients. Sometimes it is because they are a little short of money, but it's not the only reason.

"Sometimes it is cultural. French patients and doctors are a little more aggressive in fighting for the last months of a patient's life with new drugs."

In a total lifespan it is not much, maybe, but it can be very important in the life of a patient. It could be the most important month of their lives. I have patients who have shown no interest in their family for years, but

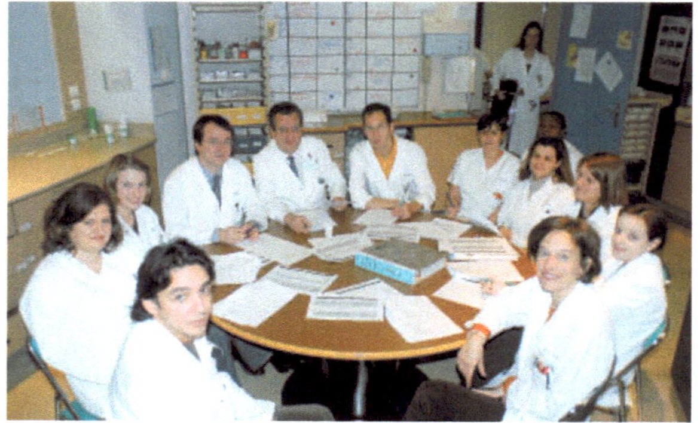

The Phase I Unit at the Institut Gustave-Roussy, Villejuif, 2003

then 3 months before they die, they see their son and daughter in a way they haven't done for 30 years. It can be a fantastic time in terms of intensity and family feeling."

At the European level, he is Chairman of the Protocol Review Committee (PRC) at the European Organisation for Research and Treatment of Cancer (EORTC) and a member of the Board. His Committee's task is to decide, with the help of international experts, on scientific quality and the feasibility of every protocol outline submitted to EORTC. Once an idea is accepted, he works with researchers to help them build a full protocol. It's a lot of work, he says, but he clearly enjoys promoting large randomised trials and helping to get them recognised at the international level.

"I can't accept that the different specialties can do their own work and ignore others."

His recent stints as Executive Medical Director of the Federation of European Cancer Societies (FECS), in 2000 and 2002, were more frustrating. Charged with the task of encouraging the six member societies to work together, he said, "I had more hope in this project than I could realise. I can't accept that the different specialties can do their own work and ignore others, but there are a lot of groups and they don't always want to work together. It's a problem."

More positively, Armand has chaired the Flims educational workshop on methods in clinical trial design for many years. Flims is an initiative sponsored jointly by FECS, the American Society of Clinical On-

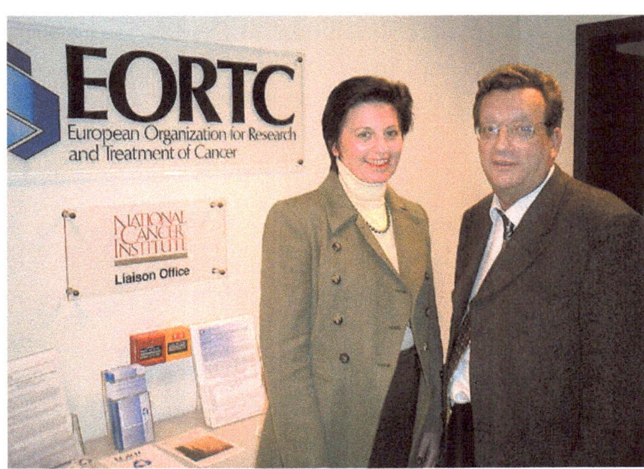

cology (ASCO) and the American Association for Cancer Research (AACR). Though it receives more money from the US than from Europe, its effect is to nurture a network of European oncologists. "Most young oncologists in Europe go the the States to improve their knowledge. When they return, they have good links with Americans, but tend to ignore their colleagues in Europe. Now, through the Flims workshop, we have a network of 400 young oncologists, who know, talk to and visit each other. There is no money behind exchanges, but young oncologists who are friends are trying to work together."

The fate of young oncologists is a preoccupation for Armand. As a young oncologist himself, in 1974, with the support of Georges Mathé, he was a founder member of the European Society for Medical Oncology (ESMO). He was later a member of its scientific committee for many years, and President in the early 1990s. But his early introduction to the international scene gave the young intern a terrific boost and was indicative of the opportunities available at the time. Ironically, for one

With Françoise Meunier, head of the EORTC, where he chairs the Protocol Review Committee, 2003

so much part of the fabric of European oncology, he is concerned that existing structures are stifling the specialty and making it less attractive to young doctors.

"Oncology is now so well organised and structured, with an archbishop and bishops and so on, that it is no longer an open field."

"When I entered oncology in France, it was a totally empty field. We had good surgeons and radiotherapists, but there were no medical oncologists; the specialty did not exist. I had the pleasure of being one of the first generation of oncologists and participating in the development of oncology. We were very enthusiastic; there weren't many of us but we were friends throughout France and Europe. It's a little funny that 30 years later, when there is a lot of work to do, the opportunities for young oncologists are not as great and they are not as enthusiastic as we were. Oncology is now so well

organised and structured, with an archbishop and bishops and so on, that it is no longer an open field. It is blocked and that is not optimal for the young oncologist."

"The freedom we had years ago in oncology still exists in neuropsychology, and that's where you find enthusiastic young people. It is not the same throughout Europe; countries that developed oncology later than France, such as Spain, still have enthusiastic young people. But in France this is not the case. We have too much control over our young doctors, we should be more confident in them than we are."

So would Armand enter oncology if he were starting out today? Yes, he says, but he would try to find a way other than through the official channels. There are appealing possibilities now in pharmacogenetics, which did not exist then, and openings now are "much more scientific than political," he says.

Armand has become part of European oncology, but, years ago, it was not at all obvious that this is

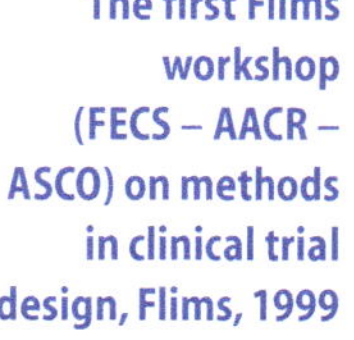

The first Flims workshop (FECS – AACR – ASCO) on methods in clinical trial design, Flims, 1999

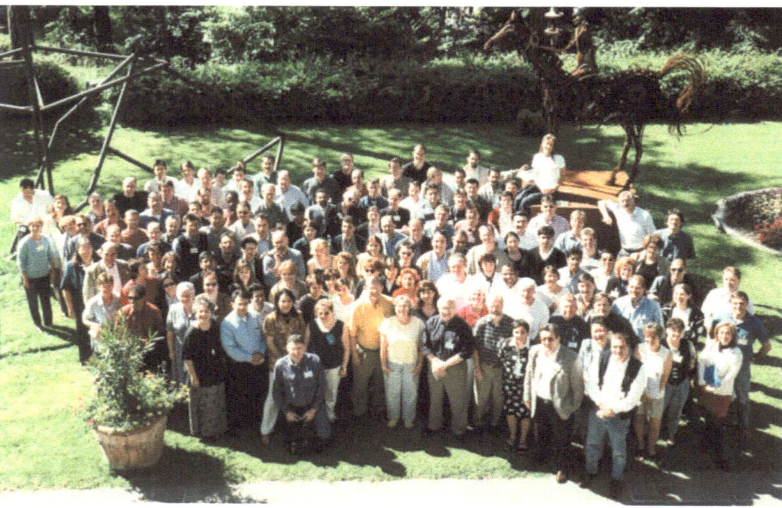

where he would end up. His family's roots are in Auvergne, a poor area in central France. But while the family retains its links – Armand has a house there – for generations they have had to move to find work. Armand was born and brought up in Algeria where his father, a civil servant, was working for the French government.

He was fascinated by the country and the culture, even learning Arabic at school, while his French friends went for English or German. He delighted in being the only French boy in a class of 25 Arab students. It helped him understand more deeply the country where he was living, as well as, perhaps, satisfying a desire to be different, and taking a different path from his contemporaries. He stayed in Algeria until he was 15, and relished it. He says the experience opened his mind to different civilisations and cultures; reading, learning about them and visiting, has become a lifelong interest.

Armand's family is not medical – he is the only doctor – and he would have been happy to study ethnology at university. But he plumped for medicine, more because it allowed him to delay his final career decision and perhaps hold on to his cherished freedom a bit longer – medical students can become psychiatrists, researchers, work for a pharmaceutical company, or whatever.

Pre-clinical medicine bored him so much that he chose to study homeopathy and acupuncture alongside it.

Partly driven – again – by the desire to be different, he was marking time until his studies became more

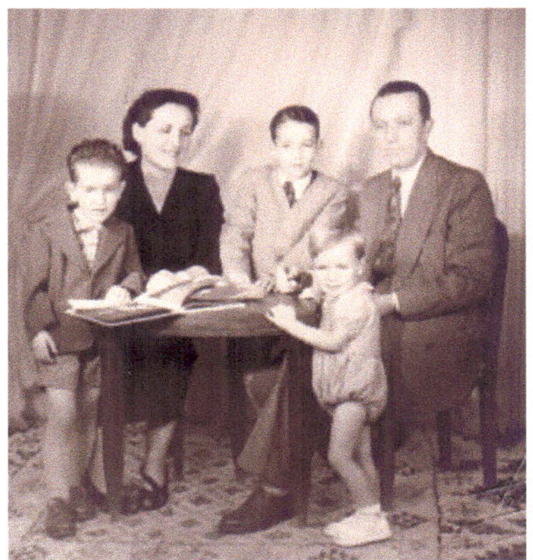

The eldest of three sons. The Armand family in Algeria, 1952

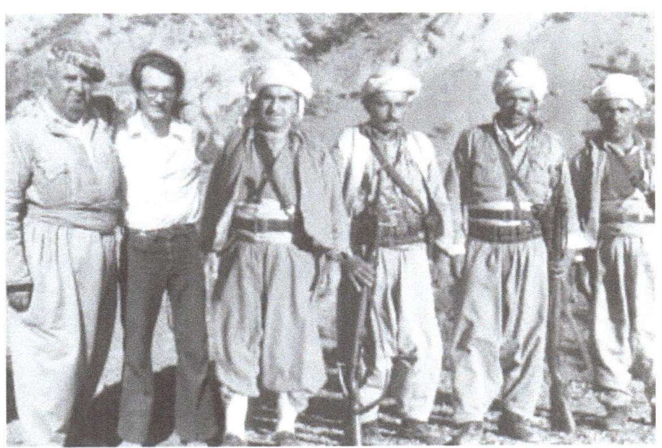

interesting. He was never convinced by homeopathy, but can converse on the subject with a knowledge rare in mainstream medicine. And then, of course, there were his hitchhiking tours in the long summer vacations. It was the perfect way to travel, not only because he was a cash-strapped student, but because it made him depend on and relate to the local people, and get to know their country from the inside. For months each year he was free to roam across Greece and Turkey, Iraq (where in 1970 he was close to General Barzani, head of the Kurdish revolt against Saddam Hussein), Syria and Israel. He is almost wistful as he remem-

With General Barzani and his Kurdish Peshmerga in Iraq in 1972

bers: "I had time, and that's a big difference from now. Plenty of time. I was so rich with this freedom. I do not enjoy my travelling today in the same way."

By the end of his third year, medicine was interesting him more, and he decided to forego his travelling to spend a month in London one summer, at the orthopaedic department of the London Hospital (now the Royal London) in Whitechapel. Bizarrely, his professor, Sir Reginald Watson Jones, mistook a rather pronounced French accent for that of a cockney, but Armand was pleased to be understood and set about making international friends in medicine, some of whom later went into oncology.

> **"I felt that if I didn't take the opportunity to do something different, my life would be unchanged for the next 20 years in Toulouse."**

He was always on the lookout for opportunities to get off the beaten track. After qualifying from Toulouse, where by that time his family was living, he was obliged to do his military service. He could have worked at a military hospital in Toulouse, as most young doctors wanted, but, "I felt that if I didn't take the opportunity to do something different, my life would be unchanged for the next 20 years in Toulouse. Everyone was looking for a job in the local hospital. But I wanted to leave and go somewhere with a different culture. I took some extra training and went to Nepal."

He stayed for two years as head of the haematology laboratory in Kathmandu. He enjoyed the work and, while there, was offered a position with the World Health Organization, working for the health system of Tibet. It was tempting, but pragmatism prevailed: "If I had stayed, I would have had to drop clinical and scientific research, which was the one field I had not made the most of. So I came back."

It wasn't easy, since returning meant trading authority and opportunities for becoming an ambitious young doctor stuck back in the French system. But within months he was off again, this time to Columbia University, New York. He worked in immunology, on a project investigating whether addictive drugs such as heroin and cannabis could change immunological status. It was a heady time. He had a paper published in Science for the first time, and made friends with fellow researchers from all over the world. The addicts were interesting, the work productive, and as for the American way of life: "When I was in Tibet, or Nepal, I was much closer to understanding the people there, what they were doing and what their aims were, than to the amusing specimens of fauna in New York. For me, it was a totally

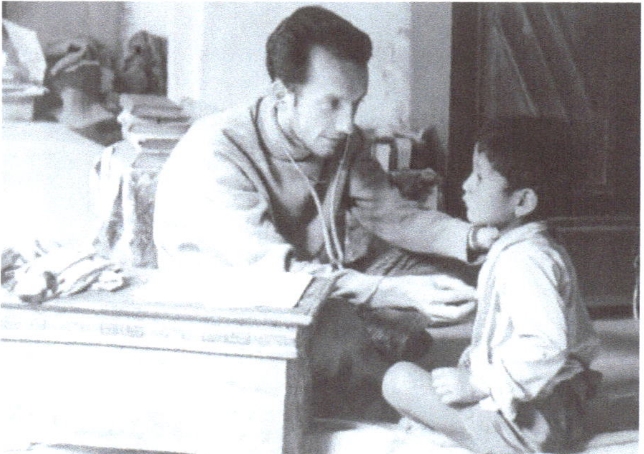

wild country, but the discovery was fantastic."

Again, he considered staying on, possibly indefinitely. But the lure of France was great, despite having lived elsewhere for most of his life at that point. He returned and entered oncology, rather to the surprise of his peers. "It had a poor status at the time.

"People seemed to think I was choosing to be some kind of voluntary worker, taking care of dying people."

That was not the case at all. I like to take care of patients even if they are in a difficult situation, but we did have the chance to do something for them – that was not seen by many people then."

"Oncology also allowed you to remain an internist, and take care of patients in their totality. In the 1970s, organ-oriented specialties were developing: nephrologists, cardiologists, and though this was technically successful, it was too limiting for me. The global specialty of cancer with cancer patients appealed much more. And it was an open field.

"There was a lot of nepotism in medicine at the time and a lot of opportunities were sewn up by the son-of-Mr-So-and-So."

Not the daughter.
"It was the right decision. I would do the same again."
The 1970s was a good time in medicine. There was money for research, hospitals were being built, everything was possible. He was in at ground level in European oncology,

a founding member of ESMO shortly after his return from the States, and seems to have been in the right place at the right time. The field was open, he was asked by Maurice Tubiana to move from Toulouse to Paris, and built the Phase I Unit, and the career that he wanted.

He still exudes enthusiasm, both for his own work and oncology in general. For example, he has just embarked on an institutional project to arrange collaboration with small start-up companies who have drugs but little knowledge of phase I development. Partnerships will be established so that the Institut Gustave-Roussy carries out the phase I work, but both benefit financially through shared patents from the success of any future drugs. Armand is effusive. "It's a fantastic new challenge and quite different from what I could imagine when I started my career in the 1970s."

Oncology itself is set to change radically in the next five years, he predicts. "We will have access to active treatments we cannot even imagine today. Two years ago, I was

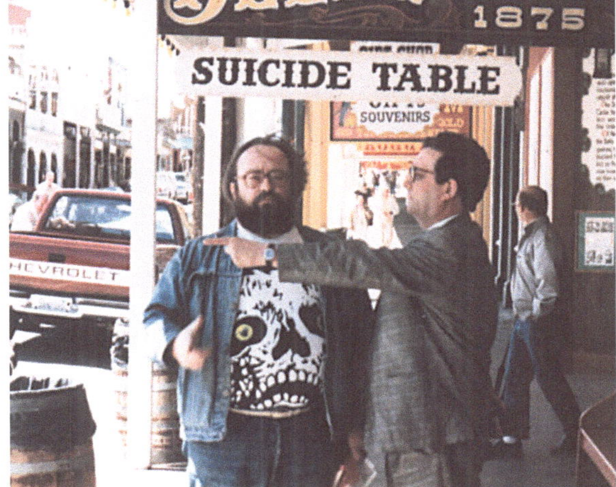

In Reno, Nevada, with his friend Esteban Cvitkovic, with whom he worked for nine years at the Institut Gustave-Roussy 3, Savigny-le-Temple, 1992

not as confident of this as I have become. Now it is clear that the oncology of the future will be different because of the tools we have for the patient and, because of this, the organisations we need. We will have a new nosology of the different cancers based on genomics. The classical prognostic TNM staging system (primary tumour – regional lymphnodes – distant metastasis) invented by Pierre Denoix from the Institut Gustave-Roussy will be radically modified. We may not need cancer centres for intensive therapeutic approaches.

"Except for the diagnosis and global strategy, we may see treatments that are accessible to general physicians. Radiotherapy and chemotherapy could be given locally."

It's almost as if oncology itself is about to complete its first full circle, from local care, through the development of the specialist team and specialist centre, and back to local care, this time with a backing of knowledge and expertise previously unknown. Armand has seen the cycle through, and it has been thrilling.

Not that the work was done without sacrifices. The work-life balance was not for him. "Medicine was very important in my life. I cannot say it was something I did beside everything else. I was so involved in medicine, it was my life."

But it opened doors, which interested him hugely. Medical contacts in China and Asian countries led to invitations, and he was an early visitor to China in the 1970s. Most of his travelling, especially later, was related to his clinical work, and he developed interests in cancers common in the Far East. It was through one of these that he met his future wife.

Ju-Liya is a physician and immunologist, MD, PhD, Chinese with a passion for French culture. They met in Paris through a shared professional interest in naso-pharyngeal cancer (a common Chinese and North African Disease he worked on for nine years with Dr Esteban Cvitkovic). Armand says that "Of all the fantastic qualities Liya has, she is also a window on this world." She has opened up a lot of possibilities for him in China.

"It took a long time for her to become my wife," he says, but finally she did, and they now have a six-year-old daughter, Marie-Anne Yulan – her name part French, part Chinese. Armand has never managed to master the Chinese language, but his daughter is fluent not only in French and Chinese, but also in Arabic, taught by her nanny. One of his

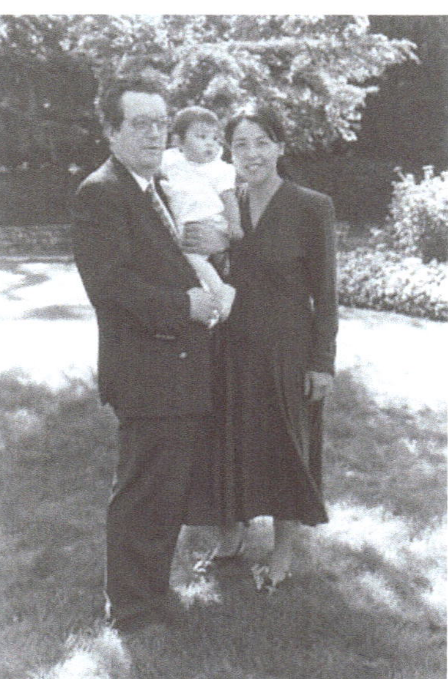

Cover Stories

greatest pleasures is speaking Arabic with Marie-Anne.

He swims at the pool within his apartment block and loves his wife's cooking. "She is a chemist and a fantastic cook. She cooks Chinese, she cooks French and she invents a lot of dishes which are somewhere in-between!" His wife's professional standing helps keep a sense of proportion, and when she was invited to the French Ambassador's, and he tagged along as spouse, he was amused that they were introduced to the ambassador, whom he knows, as "Dr Ju-Liya and Mr Armand".

He is now "more or less obliged" by his wife and daughter to go back to Auvergne more often. He has taken his house for granted, as a place for future partial retirement, not to live in now. "I was not close to this place and I wanted to go to other countries. But my wife and my daughter have become involved in projects. My wife visits China every month; even so, she is developing a plant programme in the middle of

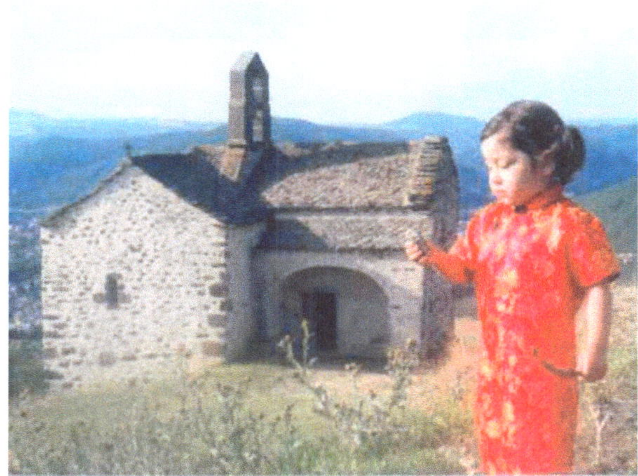

Marie-Anne in Cantal, Auvergne

Auvergne. She is much more socially active there than I am."

The traveller is finally, literally, putting down roots and building an arboretum in Auvergne. There already are trees of more than 100 years in age; some apple trees are 150 years old. Every year, Armand and his wife plant trees with their daughter. He brings olive trees and fig trees from southern Europe, which remind him of Algeria. She brings trees from her native China. "My family has been there for 400 years and there were many classical trees there. But we are planting different kinds of trees with my daughter and building a family archive. In 30 or 40 years she will still have these trees. It is a way to still be here," he says.

Now approved for metastatic breast cancer in most European countries including:

Germany   France   Italy   Spain

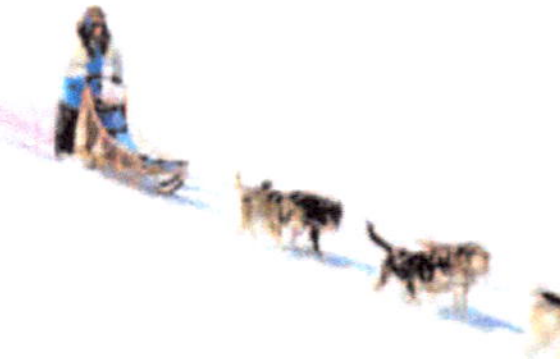

GEMZAR combined with paclitaxel

For more information, visit www.LillyOncology.com

Myelosuppression is usually the dose-limiting toxicity.

The most common grades 3/4 hematologic adverse events in patients receiving GEMZAR/paclitaxel for metastatic breast cancer are neutropenia, leukopenia, anemia, and thrombocytopenia. The most common grades 3/4 nonhematologic adverse events are alopecia, fatigue, neuropathy, liver enzyme elevation, and myalgia.

For complete product information, please refer to the SPC approved in your country.

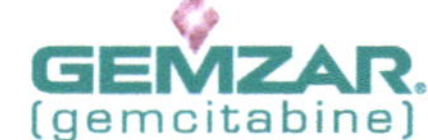

Silvia Marsoni: The Go-Between

Helen Saul

At the Southern Europe New Drug Organization (SENDO)'s most recent annual retreat, its consultant, Dr Marcel Rozencweig, complimented the team on remarkable progress since its inception in 1997. His evident surprise prompted the director, Dr Silvia Marsoni, to ask what probability SENDO's scientific mentors had given to its success at the outset. "Zero," came the reply. "Or perhaps two percent."

Less determined or, she says, more realistic, people would have faltered in the face of such odds. Not so Marsoni. She makes her choices on the basis of what she wants to do rather than on a calculated assessment of what is readily achievable. She would have gone for it, even if she had been aware of the scale of her mentor's doubts. It was a long-cherished dream, and anyway, she relishes a stab at the impossible.

Marsoni's career has been a series of five- to seven-year cycles, each involving some kind of start-up. Her projects have encompassed aspects of cancer research from early drug development to large-scale clinical trials – as well as an "accidental" stint in politics. Sometimes she comes down with a bump, but she always bounces back. The day after she was ousted from her political post, as President of Biella province, she reported for work at SENDO,

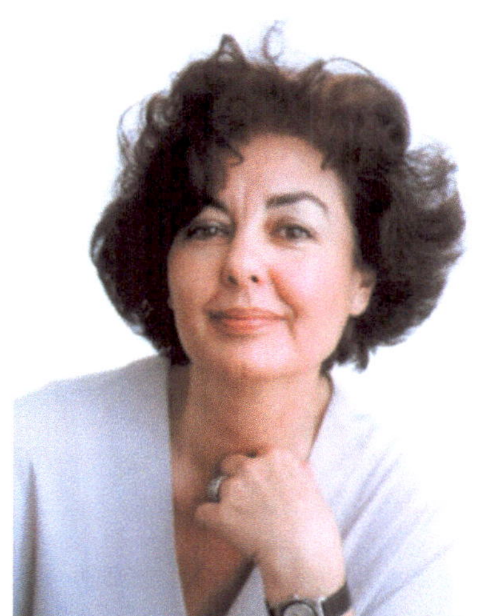

and was greeted with a champagne reception.

Biella's loss was certainly SENDO's gain. Under Marsoni's direction, it has sprung from nowhere to become a thriving enterprise. SENDO is, she says, "a one-stop shop for drug development." It is a network of networks, and she, at the hub, coordinates work in clinics, hospital laboratories, basic research centres involving molecular biology and animal systems, and so on. It is her job to round up the heads of various centres in Milan and Switzerland and make them work together. "Once a project is decided on, I provide the stroma that links the centres together so that they can

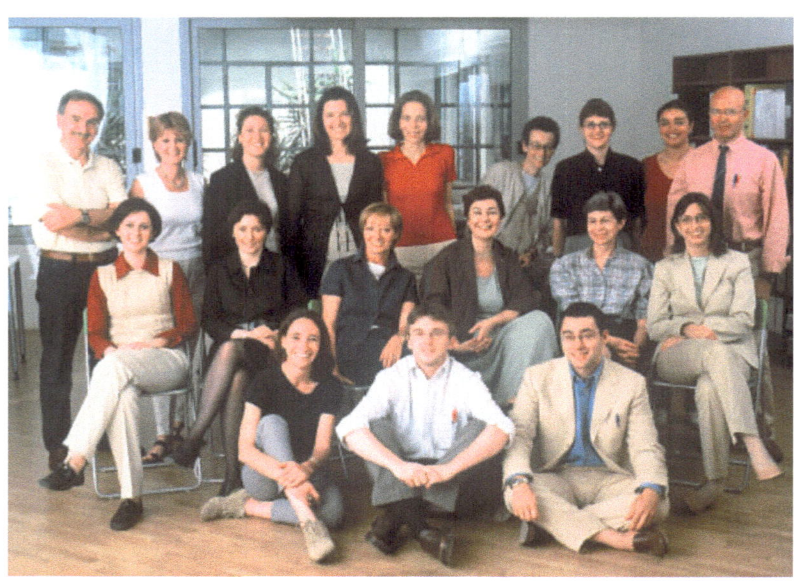

The SENDO team

produce ideas. Then I take the ideas and turn them into reality."

SENDO has grown out of the friendship between five medical students at the University of Milan in the 1970s. Marsoni, Cristiana Sessa, Luca Gianni, Maurizio D'Incalci, and Raffaella Giavazzi. By the time they were in their early 40s, all but Sessa (in Switzerland) were working in their own area in Italy, and becoming dissatisfied with what they were able to achieve. Drugs for early clinical research were scarce in Italy at the time, partly because of the prevailing view that drug development could safely be left to industry; partly because the Italian Ministry of Health had a baroque and circumlocutory way of handling dossier filing, which meant that a procedure which took 15 days in Switzerland or 45 days in the UK could take anywhere between a few months and many years in Italy. "Industry wouldn't touch Italy with a barge pole," said Marsoni.

No drugs in early clinical research meant none in late clinical research or phase III trials either, since the groups involved in the early stages tend to go on to develop the drugs further. In addition, there was, and is, little public funding for clinical research in Italy. All of which was extremely frustrating for the friends. At the time Marsoni was designing phase III trials, D'Incalci was in preclinical research, as was Giavazzi, who had a particular interest in angiogenesis. Sessa was running phase I trials and Gianni, high-tech phase II/III trials.

"Once a project is decided on, I provide the stroma that links the centres together so that they can produce ideas. Then I take the ideas and turn them into reality."

They decided that the only way to gain access to new drugs would be to set up a mechanism for early clinical research. With support from Dr Alberto Costa, Director of the European School of Oncology, they eventually found funds, from the FIRC (Fondazione Italiana per la Ricerca sul Cancro) and the National Cancer Institute in the US. They then faced the even trickier task of establishing themselves as a unit in a city that already possessed six or seven major cancer institutes. Enter the Swiss lymphoma specialist and politician, Franco Cavalli, who enticed Professor Umberto Veronesi, at the European Institute of Oncology, Professor Silvio Garattini, at the Mario Negri, and Professor Franco Rilke at the Istituto Nazionale dei Tumori, to join the project.

Cavalli was interested in working with a group with access to a larger patient base and SENDO was an opportunity for him too, thus his intervention was entirely welcome and led, in 1997, to the foundation of SENDO.

At the time, that meant Marsoni, a couple of part-time assistants and a secretary sitting in a room. But it was never going to remain that way for long. "It was therapeutic for me, because I had just had such a set-back with politics. I was back in my own field and I was determined to make it. I am single-minded and passionate." Banking on her past experience as "drug developer" at the National Cancer Institute in Bethesda and calling up all her own and her colleagues credits in the field SENDO was created and "sold" to the pharmaceutical world. Competition was, and remains, fierce but challenges have never daunted some one like Marsoni.

The attitude has borne fruit. SENDO is now a 17-person hub, lin-

king centres throughout Italy and Switzerland, and part of the European Drug Development Network. It is based in a converted garage in the centre of Milan, all huge open spaces, immensely high ceilings, wooden floors and glass/metal partitions. The space was derelict when Marsoni first saw it, but she has a long-standing interest in industrial architecture and recognised its potential immediately. She oversaw renovations that retained the character of the building and include plans for a third floor roof garden in the next phase. "Everybody loves working in this building," she says. It would be hard not to.

> "It was therapeutic for me,
> because I had just had such a
> set-back with politics.
> I was back in my own field and
> I was determined to make it."

A typical chain of events in a SENDO project starts with a brain storming within the team, then everybody sets forth with his/her own specific "homework" according to their own competences. Typically Gianni does the trial design. Marsoni makes a synopsis of it, and discusses it with Sessa. If Sessa, who probably has more phase I experience than anyone else in Europe, believes it is realistic, Marsoni takes it back to Gianni. He designs the pharmacology parts, which are then taken to D'Incalci to see if it works in an animal system, and the results, positive or negative, go back to Gianni for further discussion. Marsoni says, "I link people and I link ideas. I take ideas and make them work."

On top of this, SENDO offers the services of a commercial research organisation to industry: data management, clinical and medical monitoring, filing with regulatory agencies and ethical committees, organising meetings with investigators, arranging the arrival of drugs. As a result, the bulk of its funding now comes directly from industry, on a fee per service basis. The rest is from private foundations, government grants, charities and so on.

"I link people and I link ideas. I take ideas and make them work."

Marsoni wants SENDO to be able to work with academia, not just industry, to develop compounds. "We can not leave drug development solely in the hands of industry, because it is there, let's not ever forget it, to make money out of drugs. It is not a charity. It needs good drugs in order to do this, but once a drug is on the market, a company might not be interested in opening up new areas which are not commercially rewarding. So organisations like SENDO, the European Organisation for the

Research and Treatment of Cancer, Cancer Research UK, have a mission to do their own development, even if the drugs come from industry. The world needs SENDO and SENDO-like organisations."

It's an ambitious statement, given that only a few years ago, even its backers gave SENDO little chance of success. But Marsoni is not one to shrink from a challenge. Right from the beginning, she studied medicine against the wishes of her father, who thought she would be better off getting married, and didn't understand anyway why she wanted to look after sick people. "He was very conventional and very Italian," Marsoni says. For two years she worked to pay her own way through university, but was struggling. He finally agreed to help her, as long as she got top class grades and graduated six months early. She agreed to his conditions and then achieved them.

Her background was "privileged" says Marsoni. "I consider myself a fortunate person, I have been given a lot from life." She certainly has influential forebears and it's been quipped that she and her husband Francesco, a philosopher and aristocrat, between them have family members who played a part in most of the key events of Italian history. For example, her home town, Biella, is a textile town, home of the industrial revolution in Italy. An ancient relative of Marsoni's mother was instrumental in this development; he went to England to learn and import the mechanical skill of weaving. Mills and factories were built on the edges of the river in Biella, from the 17th century, right up to the turn of the 20th century. Now abandoned, they still make a dramatic feature on

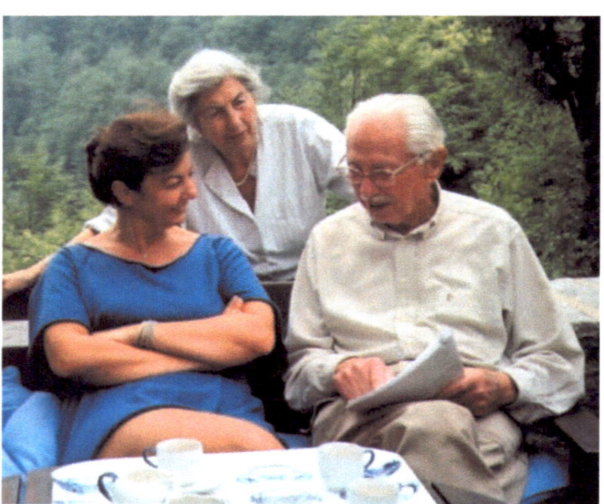

the landscape, and probably shaped Marsoni's love of such architecture. Biella's textiles have made it to the heart of current affairs: the town is home to Ermenegildo Zegna, notably the manufacturer of the tie that Monica Lewinsky gave to Bill Clinton.

"We can not leave drug development solely in the hands of industry, because it is there, to make money out of drugs. It is not a charity."

Then there is a famous Renaissance architect, a key banker who became prime minister in the mid 19th century (and balanced the books in Italy for five years, no mean feat), and the sort of Crimean soldier who has streets in Milan named after him. Marsoni, or Silvia Marsoni married Mori Ubaldini degli Alberti Lamarmora, as it says in her passport, is steeped in Italian history.

It's been quipped that she and her husband, between them have family members who played a part in most of the key events of Italian history.

Her personal history is also colourful. She grew up in Venice, her father's home town, and had a huge amount of freedom in a city without cars. Then, when she was 12 years old, her mother was determined to finish her education and become a psychoanalyst. This entailed moving the family to Biella, her home town, so that she could commute to Milan to study. The commute proved difficult, so the family moved again, to Milan. Four years later, her mother finished her education in Milan and

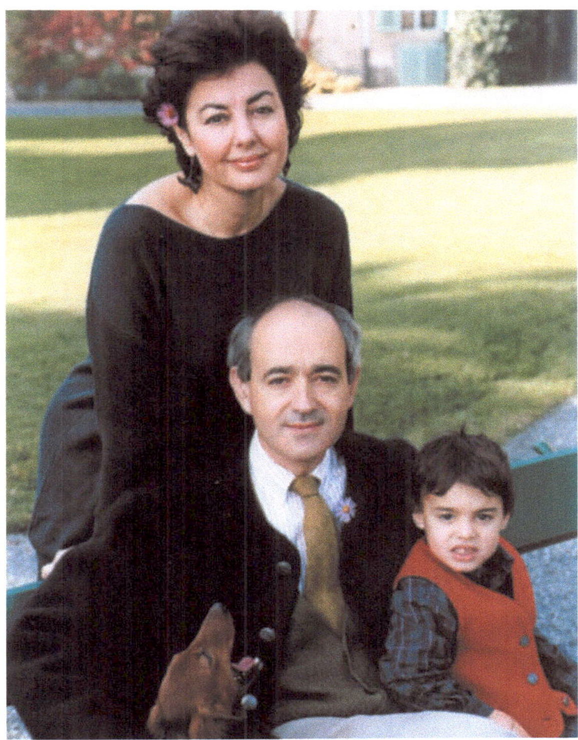

decided to complete her training at the Tavistock Institute in London. "If you think I am single-minded, she is 100 times more so. Nothing stands in her way, she runs over any obstacle!"

The only thing that Marsoni regrets, in an interesting and varied career, is that she did not go with her mother then, and complete her own education in England. She was in her last year at high school, heavily involved in the revolution of the early 1970s, and decided to stay in Milan with her father. Her brother, who is four years younger, did; he became an architect and has stayed in London ever since. Interestingly, Marsoni says that if she had her time again, she would have chosen to be an architect too.

Family portrait, with dog Valdi, in the garden of the family house in Biella

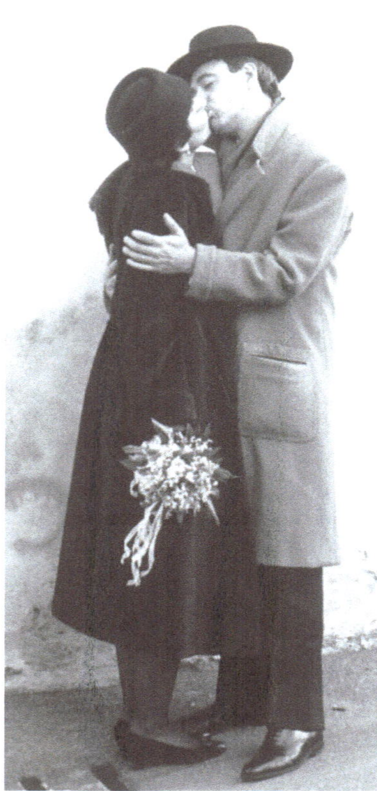

The kiss

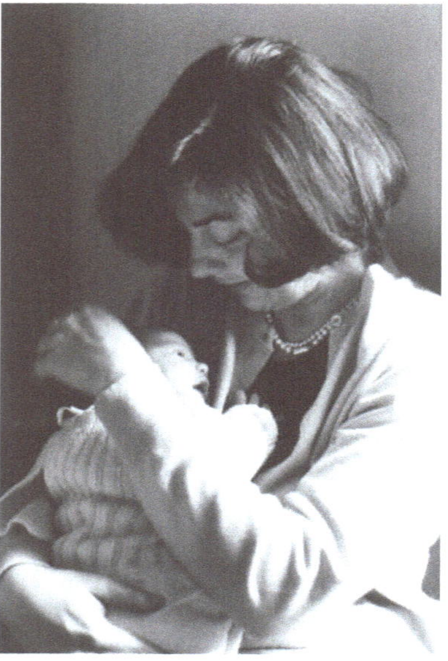

The first day

Anyway, Marsoni sailed through university, and had chosen her specialty by her third or fourth year, when she went to the Mario Negri. "I had no doubt about cancer, perhaps because it deals with systems which are not repairable. Or maybe it is like love. You become interested in one person and not in another, who really is just as nice."

Whatever. It was always going to be cancer for Marsoni and, soon after qualifying, she read a pivotal paper on clinical trials by Richard Peto at Oxford University. "It changed my life. I knew as I read it that this is what I wanted to do." She was unable to go to Peto's lab in Oxford but decided to stay and set up large clinical trials in Italy. Her first attempt, in non-small cell lung cancer (NSCLC), she describes as "horrendous". "I was seriously proud of it, but it had five arms and was a totally inappropriate design and sample size – all the kinds of things that suggest that, actually, I must not have read the Peto paper properly at all!"

Marsoni is disarmingly open about past failures. She studies them, dissects them almost, and learns whatever she can from them. She comes across as exuberant, outgoing and confident. Her penchant for going for whatever she wants, without considering its feasibility, has meant that some ideas have had to mull for a decade or more before anything comes of them. Large-scale clinical trials were one such. Having just decided that this was what she was going to devote her career to, she was offered a fellowship to the National Cancer Insitute in the US. And off she went to work in early drug development – almost the opposite end of the research spectrum.

Marsoni is disarmingly open about past failures. She studies them, dissects them almost, and learns whatever she can from them.

She loved the US and settled in immediately. While her compatriots felt homesick and yearned for Italian coffee, she never looked back. She loved the physical space in the US; even the National Institute of Health campus felt right. "At the time there were fewer buildings than there are now, and it was physically beautiful, like being in the middle of a field. And there were Lyriodendrum tulipifera all over the place. My grandfather was a botanist and was enthusiastic about this type of plant. When I was young, we would play a game, spotting these plants all over Italy, where they are very rare. So when I arrived and they were all over, I thought 'Wow, here I come, this is my place!' In the first few weeks, I was working in a lab with an outside view, and one evening, I was watching the sunset through the window, and I felt on top of the world, that I could do whatever I wanted. It was marvellous."

She grabbed the opportunities offered, and by the time she left, was Chief of the Drug Development Branch. Her interest was in the methodology of screening molecules, rather than in any particular drug. "I have always been interested in uncovering mechanisms, constructing

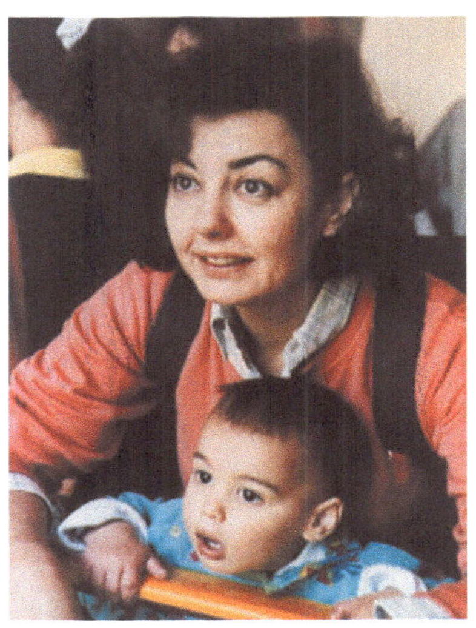

With two-year-old son Adriano, now aged 14

models to make life simpler and to help us understand reality."

The search for creative new ways of doing things and "adding a little drop of knowledge to the general body of clinical pharmacology" occupied her for almost six years. She was starting to think of going back into the clinic full-time, when a conversation with Alessandro Liberati, another Italian and former Mario Negri graduate, prompted a U-turn. It took one year, but eventually Liberati convinced Marsoni that they should go back to Italy to apply what they had learnt in the US. It was a moral and idealistic decision, based on the feeling that they could not participate in the brain drain from Europe.

"I have always been interested in uncovering mechanisms, constructing models to make life simpler and to help us understand reality."

Life in the US had been good for Marsoni; there were lots of love

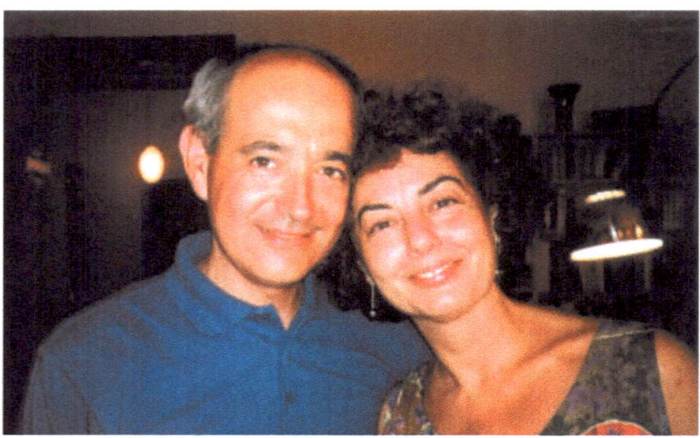

With husband Francesco

affairs, including with the architecture. It was here that she first saw and was impressed by renovated factories and warehouses in Baltimore and Montreal. But she was still single at this time, and, though it was a wrench to leave, she agreed with Liberati and back they both came. Liberati had been working on clinical trials meta-analysis, and public health issues at Harvard, Boston. So, together, they set up the laboratory of clinical pharmacology of anti-cancer drugs at the Mario Negri.

Marsoni wanted to continue developing drugs, but "it was clear after the first few months that the things I was thinking of doing were not going to be immediately feasible in Italy, because the organisation of hospitals and laboratories could not support it. The project was impractical at the time. Not impossible, because here I am, in my own drug development office. But it took 15 years to set up."

Meanwhile, she re-visited her previous fascination with Richard Peto's work and, with Liberati, set up cooperative groups to conduct large scale, phase III trials in Italy. There were lots of problems to be overcome, but they did it. It is standard practice now, but 15 years ago

they had to fight to find money, to find people, and to show that these trials could be conducted. "Things that are now considered matter-of-fact met serious resistance then, but we more than set up these trials, we introduced a mentality."

Marsoni and Liberati worked together for almost a decade, during which Marsoni also married Francesco, and had a son, Adriano. She also advanced her architectural ideas and, with a group of friends and an architect, converted a disused record factory into a highly fashionable complex of houses and flats in Milan.

"Things that are now considered matter-of-fact met serious resistance then, but we more than set up these trials, we introduced a mentality."

But in the early 1990s, Liberati felt that it was time to move on. For Marsoni, this was like undergoing a divorce, and it meant that she, too, was looking for a new challenge.

It came from an unexpected direction. Italy in the early 1990s was in the middle of the so-called tangentopoli, or bribesville, when repeated scandals led the population to reject established politicians. Professionals – scientists, clinicians, lawyers, and so on – were asked to stand for election, and Marsoni was asked to run for office in her home region of Biella. "It is a very right-wing region and I was representing the left, so my chances of being elected were zero, but they didn't have anyone else. They asked me just to give them a month of my time for the campaign, and that would be it. But I won."

Despite her earlier brush with politics as a teenager, Marsoni insists she was politically naive when she took office. She set about attempting "evidence-based politics, rather than the line-your-own pockets politics that was more common at the time," she says. Hers was a new province, recently split off from an established province, which meant there was no "machine" for her to take over. It was yet another start-up from scratch.

She spent the first three months visiting Italy, France and Switzerland to look at the models of government they were using. She gathered ideas and came back, built a team and got to work. Her stint in politics was one of the most interesting periods of her life, she now says. "It is certainly the one that taught me most about life and human beings, groups and reactions."

It was a steep learning curve. Marsoni hired 150 people in four years and ran a non-bureancratic machine. For most of her staff, this was also a first experience in politics, and the determination to do things differently was palpable. One of her greatest achievements was in the preservation of territory. Biella is a mountainous province and she came to power in the aftermath of a flood which had disrupted many of the roads. She took a typically scientific approach, made a map of risk and a map of need and where risk and need coincided, the area was prioritised.

But this was to ignore political considerations, and she failed to sell what she was doing to her electorate. "I said, scientifically, this is the area of greatest need, you have to understand it. But people do not understand through logic and fact analysis, they understand through sentiment and prejudice. My attitude was that I would not take any notice of prejudice. But a prejudiced vote counts as much as one based on illuminated thought. I was naive to think that just because I am intelligent and a scientist, trying to do things right and with a passion, that this alone would convince everyone. You have to work with prejudice and not be judgemental. If you want to be a good politician and do evidence-based government, you have to get people on your side."

In the end, the political tide was turning and Berlusconi's people swept to power in the next elections. There is little that Marsoni could have done to prevent her "demise", but she says her refusal to bow to the demands of some special interest groups was a contributor. She has been asked to return, but won't, feeling that politics is dogged by vested interests, and conflicts of interest and is not sufficiently directed towards finding the best solutions to problems.

She took a typically scientific approach, made a map of risk and a map of need and where risk and need coincided, the area was prioritised.

Nevertheless, most of her plan for the territory is being implemented by her opponents, and will start to bear fruit over the next decade or so, which is gratifying. Further, the experience has been invaluable at SENDO, where her role has been as networker extraordinaire.

Recently, Marsoni has recruited people to take over most of her exis-

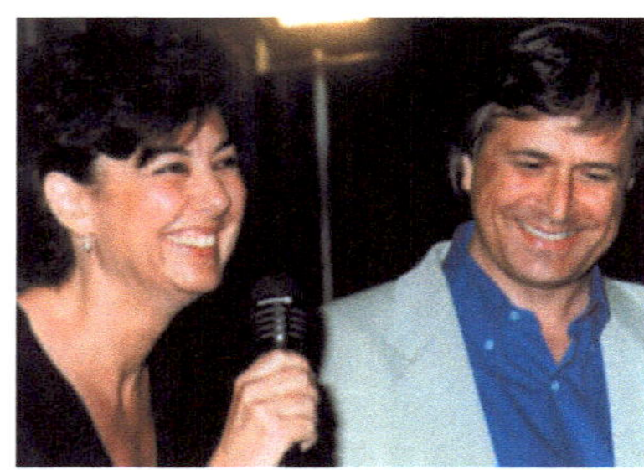

Addressing a rally with the Mayor of Cossato, Sergio Scaramal, May 1999

ting tasks, and for the next couple of years she will be devoting herself to linking up with small biotechnology companies. Most of Big Pharma now knows SENDO, but she wants to take the organisation to academia and smaller firms in the suburbs. "If an academic thinks he has found something, he goes out and sets up his own small biotech company, which is one way of doing things. He might have a talent for business, but not necessarily so. SENDO can help. I am trying to act as a go-between, bringing together the discoverer and investors, providing through SEN-DO the know-how to strike a deal, so

that everyone is happy and a potential new drug is given a chance."

One such project is already underway, in which SENDO has teamed up with a group that is half academic and half small biotech. It's a two- to three-year project, with interesting compounds and an innovative approach, and it is her "test tube", Marsoni says. "If it works, we'll just have to let it be known through the grapevine and then people will come flocking to us."

She has been asked to return, but won't, feeling that politics is not sufficiently directed towards finding the best solutions to problems

It is a crunch time for SENDO, and Marsoni believes the next year will determine whether its future can be as the "bright star" she envisages, rather than something rather more mundane. She believes that SENDO has reached its optimum size and cannot grow further without risking its capacity for informal communication. "We need to focus on phase I and early phase II trials, because this organisation requires extreme flexibility and creativity in order to function in a field in which you are bound by regulatory authorities to be extremely formal."

"I am trying to act as a go-between, bringing together the discoverer and investors..."

SENDO Milan is Italian-Swiss, but this year will see the launch of a SENDO-Spain collaboration. Groups have to remain small and local, Marsoni says, so that those involved know the mechanisms, the culture

Marsoni in her capacity as President of the Province of Biella, opening a meeting on industrial architecture – one of her great passions

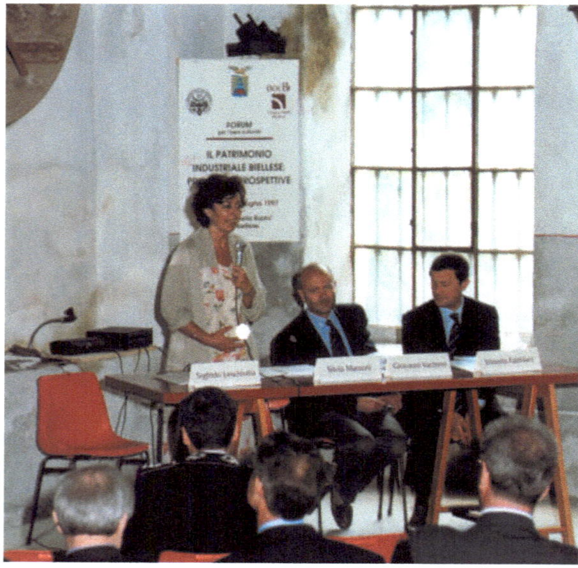

and how the group works. In five years' time, she would like to be part of a network of SENDOs throughout southern Europe. "And perhaps I can retire at this point," she says.

Marsoni? Retire? Well, not exactly. Her idea of retirement is to set up (from scratch) a restaurant in Cuba, where she has never been, but she feels would satisfy her twin loves of architecture, which is unspoilt in Cuba, and cooking. She tends to realise her dreams, so it is quite possible this will happen. But if past form is anything to go by, she has surely got time for at least one new venture before then.

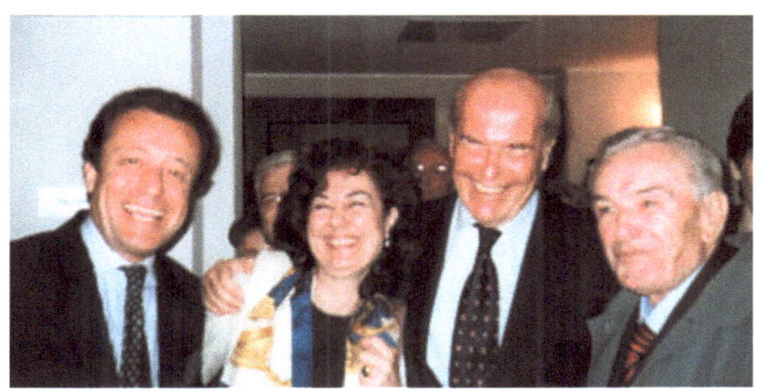

At the inauguration of the new Fondo Tempia pharmacogenomics labs in Biella, 2001. Marsoni, Alberto Costa, Director of the European School of Oncology (left), former Italian Health Minister Umberto Veronesi (right), and Elvo Tempia (far right) are all board members of the Fondo Tempia, founded in memory of son Edo Tempia, who died of melanoma

Harry Bartelink: Putting Europe First

HELEN SAUL

Professor Harry Bartelink, incoming President of the Federation of European Cancer Societies (FECS), was pensive. He had just returned from the 2003 meeting of the American Society for Clinical Oncology (ASCO), where, at the top plenary session, three of the six abstracts presented were from European groups. On the one hand, he was thinking, this demonstrates the strength of European research; on the other, it's a shame these papers were not presented and published in Europe first.

European researchers need to have more faith in their own originality, Bartelink says, and his first priority as President will be to do what he can to increase researchers' confidence and pride in their ideas and achievements. "In Europe, we have fascinating discussions between people of different countries, different traditions and cultures. The intellectual interactions between scientists are truly original," he says.

Bartelink is honoured to be President of FECS because of the Federation's unique position at the hub of the various disciplines and nationalities. "You won't find a big organisation anywhere else that has such interaction. We have everybody: surgeons, medical oncologists, radiation oncologists, paediatricians, nurses and researchers. It makes things very interesting and it's ex-

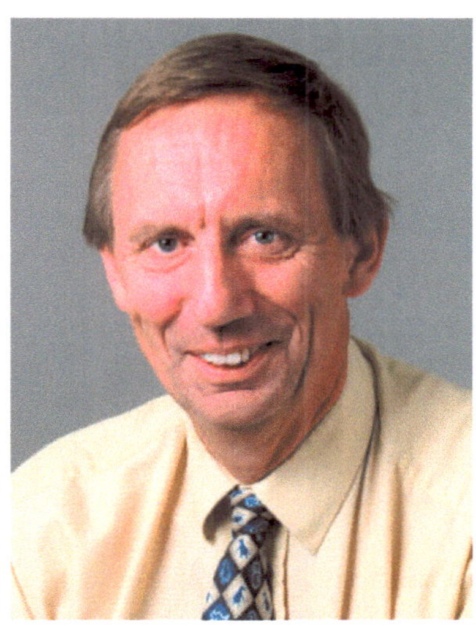

tremely important for progress in oncology. Better understanding between clinicians and researchers will open new possibilities for the future. Already in daily practice, all of us, from all the different disciplines, have to work together to offer patients the best treatment for cancer. I expect that in the coming years a lot of new opportunities will come from the improved knowledge of new targets discovered in molecular biology. For example, the exciting research of Laura van 't Veer and Marc van de Vijver in my institute has already demonstrated the powerful potential of microarrays predicting the prognosis in young breast cancer patients."

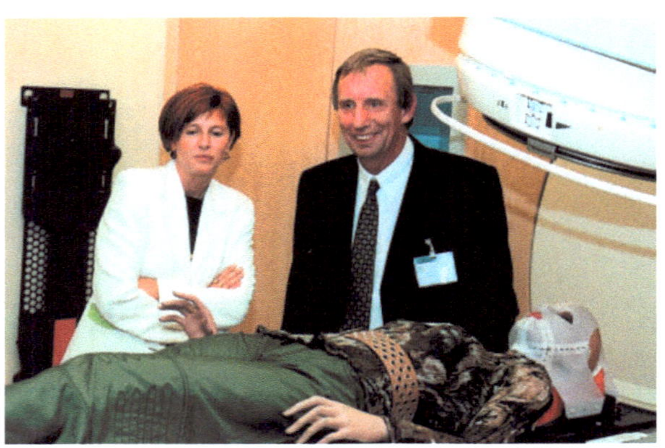

His second priority is to improve access to high-quality care for all European citizens. "The treatment that is given in Paris or Amsterdam should be available for all, wherever they live. We need quality assurance (QA) programmes to ensure that large and small hospitals everywhere offer a good quality of care." His third is to campaign for an increased budget for basic and clinical research.

Bartelink's aims may sound pretty much what you'd expect of a new President of FECS, but they are deeply rooted in the highs and lows of his own illustrious career. His own work, at Stanford University in California changed the standard treatment for lung cancer; he demonstrated that concomitant cisplatin and radiotherapy was more effective than giving the chemotherapy in advance. But he didn't vigorously pursue the initial finding on his return to Europe, leaving it to be picked up and developed in the US.

By contrast, his European work on breast cancer treatment and especially the value of QA has set the scene for his second aim and has earned him plaudits. It started as a randomised trial comparing breast conservation surgery with radical mastectomy – continuing work started in Paris and Milan – but one of the most striking findings of the study was the difference in outcomes achieved by different institutes. The local recurrence rate varied between 4 and 32%, depending on where patients were treated. In the next breast conserving therapy trial, a strict QA protocol, introduced with the support of a European Union grant, reduced the variation to between 3 and 7%.

"At the time I was shocked because the differences were enormous. We are extremely keen to implement modern molecular biology and so on, into the clinic, and we need to. But with better QA and better multidisciplinary integration, it would be fairly easy to improve survival by 10% for cancer patients in general, across Europe. That's an enormous improvement. It will take a long time for novel drugs to have the same impact."

The third aim, to increase cancer funding, grew out of a successful involvement with a campaign waged by the Dutch Society for Radiation Oncology. At one time in the Netherlands, waiting lists for radiotherapy were eight to nine weeks. "It was awful. Some patients with disease that could have been cured became incurable while they were on the waiting list. It led to a lot of tension in the department."

"...don't just accept waiting lists. Draw attention... to the situation, because things can be changed."

The campaign entailed approaching the Minister of Health

and other Members of Parliament, and informing the public that the situation was a scandal. Questions were asked in Parliament. And the campaign worked. In the past two years, radiotherapy departments in the Netherlands have seen a 30% increase in staff. The number of linear accelerators will increase from 70 in 1998 to 111 in 2005, and training opportunities for young oncologists have been expanded. "This is an example for the rest of Europe: don't just accept waiting lists. Draw the attention of the lay press and Parliament to the situation, because things can be changed," says Bartelink.

He's brimming with confidence and enthusiasm as he talks about what needs to be done, but these are big tasks. Encouraging positive interaction between disciplines is notoriously difficult. "It's not easy, but it's always fun to have a challenge. I love competition, debate and interaction, that's my nature. We all need a much better understanding of the possibilities other disciplines can offer, and that way lies progress."

He'll be working closely with FECS' executive director Kathleen Vandendael to promote FECS – and what needs to be done in oncology to involve the lay press and to politicians. There'll be initiatives such as a newsletter to keep cancer specialists up to date with advances in all fields of oncology. Existing structures such as the Flims Workshop, which brings together young people from all cancer disciplines, will focus on facilitating exchanges of fellows between different countries and different specialties. FECS is attacking problems on all fronts and Bartelink seems positively zealous as he outlines the way ahead.

It makes his early career all the more surprising. Where now he is focussed to the point of obsession, in the early years of his career, he seems to have had no clear sense of purpose at all, except for, on occasion, avoiding things he particularly did not want to do.

He chose medicine, for example, because he was "very bad" at languages at school and it seemed an ideal way of never again having to speak English, French or German. He smiles at the irony. "I am punished later," he says. He wanted to go to university at Groningen, but was placed instead at Nijmegen, and he accepted the place quite happily. He had a fantastic time as a student, and in fact met his wife there, another medical student and now a geriatrician.

Most students from Nijmegen at the time became family doctors, and Bartelink obligingly followed the same course. His practice was based near a huge abattoir, where many of his patients worked. They had low salaries, small houses and got a lot of stomach pains. "As a family doctor, I felt limited to change anything. For me, it was a disaster."

Another farewell party

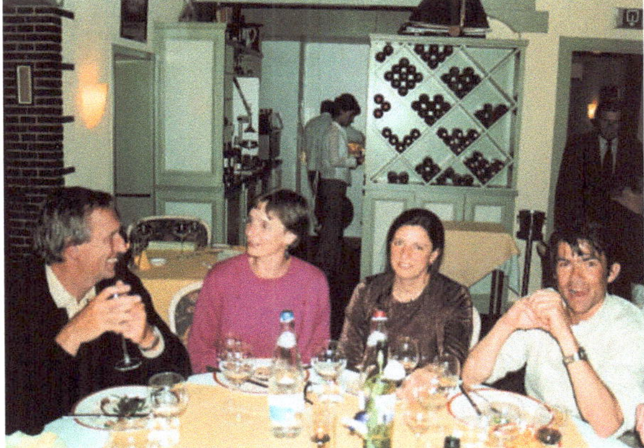

> **"I wanted to see patients that I could do something for. So the combination of this man and the possibilities led me to radiotherapy."**

During his training, he had been impressed by radiation oncologist Dirk Miete, who chaired multidisciplinary meetings in oncology. "His wisdom, his approach, his knowledge of the field – he inspired me. I thought about him when I was seeing the patients with stomach pains. I wanted to see patients that I could do something for. So the combination of this man and the possibilities led me to radiotherapy."

He was offered a training place at Nijmegen, which would have exempted him from military service, but chose instead to go to the Netherlands Cancer Institute (NKI) – on condition that the department also managed to get him an exemption. So he embarked on radiotherapy, having successfully avoided languages, ill-defined stomach complaints and the army, on the way.

But once there, he had found his niche. Growing up in eastern Holland as the second of four boys, he was always interested in physics and mathematics and the practical and technical side of things. Radiotherapy appealed for these reasons from the outset, and later, for many more. He expounds at length on the virtues of radiotherapy: the 50% of patients cured by radiotherapy, and the possibilities for palliation. "With one shot we can relieve pain, prevent fracture or spinal cord lesion." Bartelink was immediately at home in his subject.

Having said that, he continued to make career decisions for slightly off-the-wall reasons. He completed his training at NKI and was set to move back to eastern Holland to work with the radiation oncologist who had so impressed him in the first place. He refused an offer of work from the director at NKI and was about to buy a house in the woods in the east, thinking that was where he wanted to spend the rest of his life.

> **"With one shot we can relieve pain, prevent fracture or spinal cord lesion."**

But then as he and his wife happened to be visiting friends, they drove past a house being built beside a canal. As they looked at the house, the Dutch sailing team went past on the canal, practising for the Olympic games. Instantly, Bartelink conjured up a new future for himself, one in which he got home from work early in the summer and went sailing in the evening. So they abandoned the house in the woods, bought the new house and he stayed at NKI.

They lived there happily for 15 years, during which Bartelink managed his midweek sail twice. "They were two good occasions!" he says.

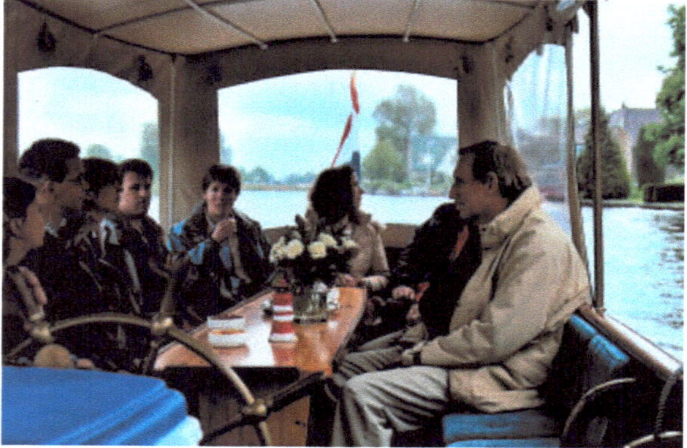

At a leaving do for a colleague at the NKI: a boat trip down the very river that had enticed Bartelink to stay and work for the Institute

The family had two boats; his four children loved sailing and took advantage of the location, even if their father didn't. It was probably the right decision, taken for somewhat over-optimistic reasons.

His career has included important stints abroad, at the Mayo Clinic (Rochester, Minnesota, USA), Institut Gustave Roussy (IGR, Paris, France) and Stanford University (Palo Alto, California, USA). In Paris in 1978, he was introduced to breast conservation surgery, when radical mastectomy was all that was on offer in Amsterdam. This led to the breast cancer project mentioned earlier.

"In some hospitals, surgery was not done according to the protocol, the tumour was not completely resected, or mammograms were not taken after surgery..."

It was a major undertaking, including 5,000 patients which, at the time, was the largest breast cancer trial ever done. It was funded by the European Union, and used a strict protocol, which outlined details of surgery, pathology, radiotherapy and radiology. This very intensive trial eliminated the large difference in outcome between institutions. Different things were going wrong in different places, he says, "In some hospitals, surgery was not done according to the protocol, the tumour was not completely resected, or mammograms were not taken after surgery to check for microcalcifications. The radiotherapy dose or distribution was sometimes not correct, or pathology not requested."

Broad cooperation across disciplines and countries enabled the project to succeed. Bartelink found little of the resistance he had expected. "It was quite amazing that people were in general very positive. They were proud to show us what they were doing, and when we made comments, nearly all changed according to our suggestions. It was much easier than I had anticipated beforehand. Of course all the centres were interested in research, but they all welcomed us. There were 38 centres in 15 countries, and afterwards they spread their knowledge throughout their own countries. So the project had a broad impact. "

At Stanford, equipment he had been promised failed to materialise. He could not embark on the project he had arrived to conduct without it and was frustrated. So he started something else altogether, looking at how best to combine chemotherapy and radiotherapy in cell lines.

Within two months, he had some encouraging results with cisplatin. He was given support from technicians and another scientist, and the work continued in mice. Daily cisplatin, given just before radiotherapy, appeared to be more effective than when a course was completed

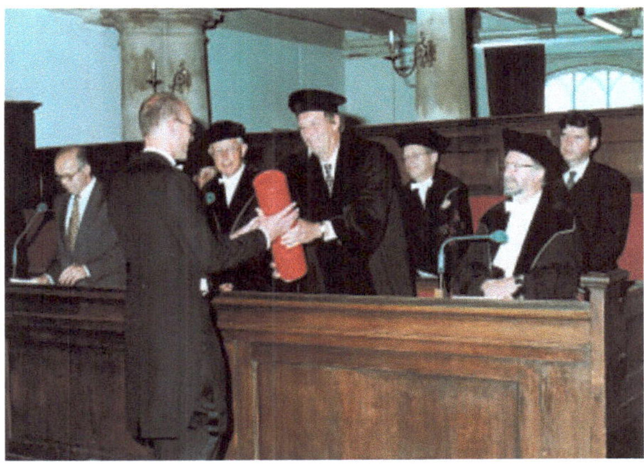

A PhD candidate has just successfully defended his thesis, and Bartelink hands him the "bul" to show he has gained his doctorate

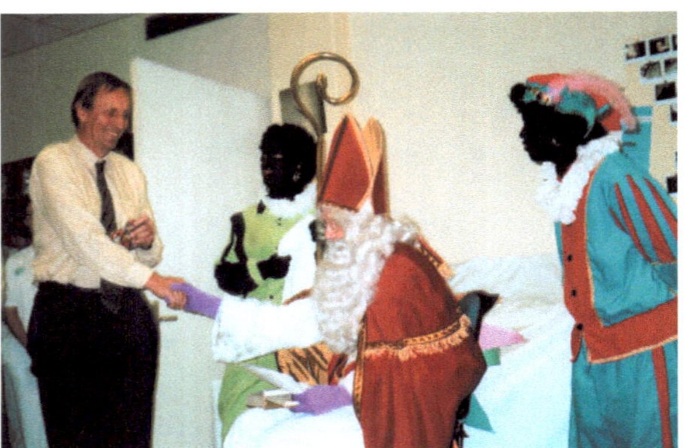

in advance of radiotherapy. On his return to Amsterdam, Bartelink set up an EORTC trial in people with lung cancer, which "to my amazement," he says, confirmed the finding in patients.

> **"It took them until 1999 to confirm that our findings were true for cervical cancer as well... Too bad that no reference was made to the initial European work!"**

This work was published in the New England Journal of Medicine in 1992, but even Bartelink was less than wholly convinced that he was on to something. "At the time I was a little bit uncertain, and perhaps suffered from the European lack of confidence, so although I continued the work to some extent, I moved most of my energy into the breast cancer work. However, our results intrigued American gynaecologists and radiation oncologists, and they tried to apply it to cervical cancer. It took them until 1999 to confirm that our findings were true for cervical cancer as well as lung cancer. Too bad that no reference was made to the initial European work!"

Bartelink had intended to stay at Stanford, but he returned when he was asked to be Chairman of the Radiotherapy Department at NKI. He and his family all loved the Californian lifestyle, but he missed European cultural and traditional diversity in academia as well as in his private life. "I learned to appreciate Europe when I was away, so when I came back I was extremely active in organisations like EORTC."

With typical pragmatism, his first task at NKI was to hire a manager to relieve him of the day to day management of the unit. It allowed him the space to oversee the strategy of his department, remain closely involved in research himself, and throw himself into European collaborations through EORTC and ESTRO.

He is especially fond of ESTRO, the European Society for Therapeutic Radiology and Oncology, and will stand down as President at ECCO in Copenhagen, when he takes up the FECS mantle. In many ways, though it's difficult to say diplomatically, he believes that ESTRO could be a model for other European cancer societies.

A key feature of ESTRO is that research in radiotherapy is not supported by pharmaceutical companies and is therefore independent. It makes setting up projects difficult, because researchers must find financial support from European or national grant-awarding bodies, but this is an advantage in the long run, Bartelink says. "We have to compete with other interests and will only get money if we have done our homework properly. Over the years we have achieved a lot of support from the EU. It means that we can look

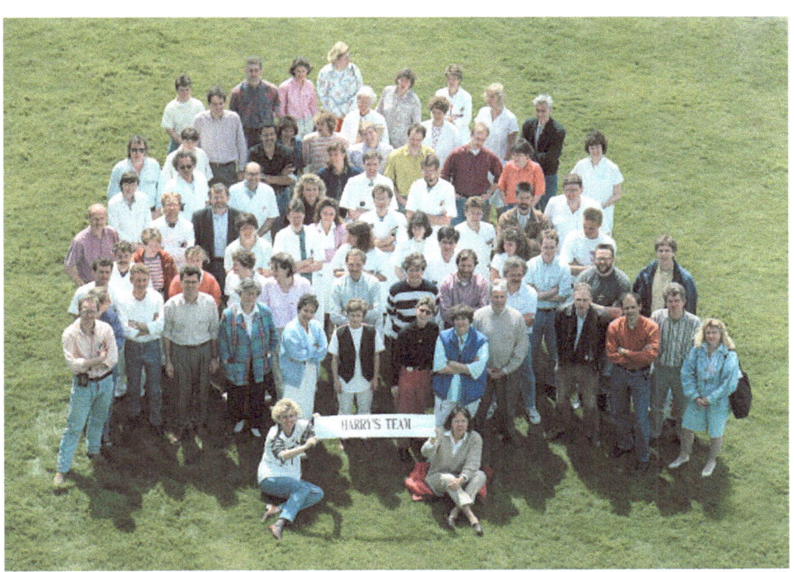

"Harry's Team" at the NKI radiotherapy department – a happening place

solely at trying to improve the treatment of cancer patients and we are not guided by the wishes of companies and their financial priorities."

"A key feature of ESTRO is that research in radiotherapy is not supported by pharmaceutical companies and is therefore independent."

ESTRO is an extremely friendly society, Bartelink says, partly because researchers are not chasing the same money. It has been effective in the key themes that Bartelink wants to focus on in his time at FECS. Training courses that bring together young radiotherapists from different countries have been running for years and have established links within the discipline throughout Europe. There is a thriving radiotherapy community in Europe, which may be one reason why Europe can claim credit for so much radiotherapy research presented for the first time – more than in any other discipline, he says. ESTRO has also worked on major QA projects, checking the facilities at different institutes, whether machines are correctly callibrated and whether appropriate doses are being given. It has been instrumental in improving standards in European radiotherapy centres, he says.

Within his own department, he is proud to have overseen work by his physicists, who developed a technique called portal imaging for linear accelerators. It allows radiotherapists to view a patient's position during treatment. The idea was sold to a US company, and the apparatus now exists all over the world. They are now cooperating with research groups in Canada and the UK to develop computed tomography-type imaging during radiotherapy. Worldwide, there are already four CT-beam accelerators now in clinical use, including one at NKI.

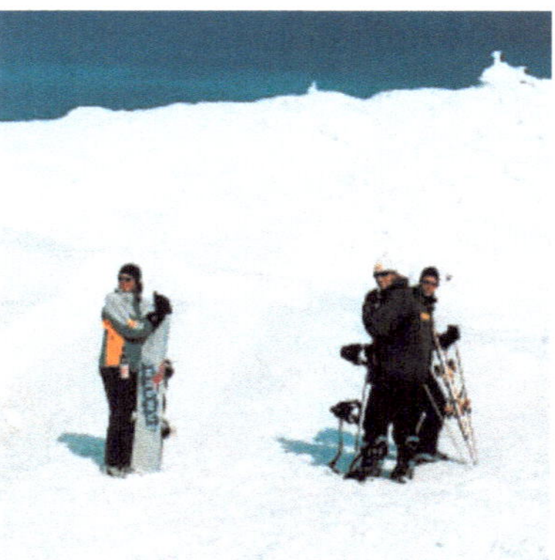

On the top of the world: on a family ski trip to Åre, Sweden

"There is a thriving radiotherapy community in Europe, which may be one reason why Europe can claim credit for so much radiotherapy research..."

His work on cisplatin and radiotherapy has been followed up within the group, and they have developed an assay that works on a smear from the buccal mucosa and predicts which patients will benefit from further treatment. "It's very nice," he says. His group is working with others in Memphis to investigate the use of a catheter to introduce cisplatin to the tumour site and irradiate simultaneously. And his radiobiologists are looking at the properties of DNA repair and how they can use it to make cells more sensitive to radiotherapy. It's a happening place.

Bartelink seems very satisfied with how his career, and indeed his life, has worked out so far, though he's slightly coy about personal details. He has many interests, but given his attempts to go sailing in the evenings, it's debatable how much time he has to devote to them. He still has a boat and sails it on the weekends. He enjoys skiing and goes on holidays with his grown-up children. And speed skating, again with the family: when the lakes are frozen in Holland, it's possible to skate for 100 km from his house. He remains close to his brothers, and the weekend after we meet he is off to his father's 84th birthday party, which sounds a big and noisy affair, attended by a host of relatives, including Bartelink senior's 13 grandchildren.

His chief interest is reading, of anything and everything, science writing to novels. And travelling, of the non-conference sort. He and his wife had planned to go to China earlier this year, to retrace a route they took 15 years ago. But their plans were scuppered by the SARS epidemic, and instead they went cycling round Provence, having a lovely, if very different, time. They've rescheduled China for next year.

In the original trip, they toured alone for five weeks using public transport, way off the beaten track. It was fascinating, he says. They spoke none of the language and had no support. Buses didn't go and they had no way of summoning help. "We have a lot of stories from that trip," he says, smiling and not telling any of them.

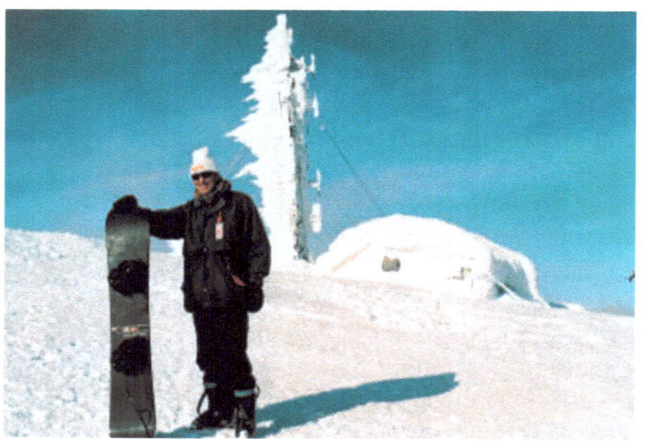

Bartelink, with two of his children, prepares to conquer Åre's mightiest peak

Nora Kearney: Shaking Up the Big House

Jim McGuigan

Nora Kearney has been called an evangelist, a maverick, a troublemaker, a visionary-depending on the viewpoint of those concerned.

In January this year she became the first nurse to be appointed to a cancer professorship in her native Scotland. It has been an eventful first 10 months, and a few boxes remain unpacked in her new office at the University of Stirling. From her desk she can see scenic Loch Airthrey and the Ochil hills reaching towards the Scottish Highlands. It is little wonder the university was recently voted the UK's most beautiful campus.

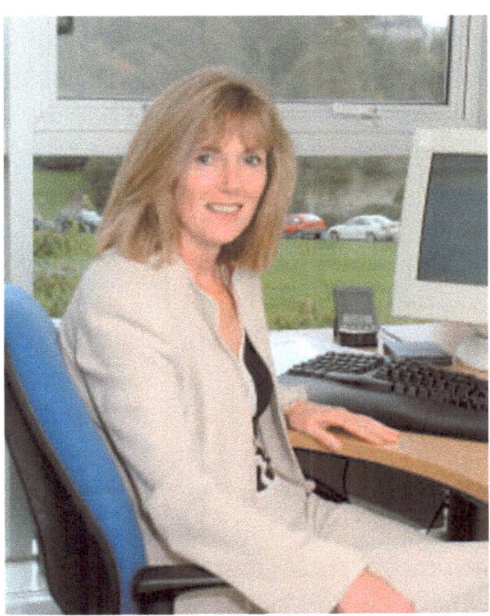

However Kearney has had little time to take in the view. Her first priority on taking up the new chair was to create a unique Cancer Care Research Centre that turns conventional thinking on its head by having the research agenda directed by patients.

In early October she was delighted to invite Scotland's Minister for Health and Community Care, Malcolm Chisholm, to open the new Centre, which his department is considering funding to the tune of £1.6 million (€2.3 million) over three years.

The new Centre is a key part of Kearney's five-year plan. Was she surprised to see it launched within her first year? "We established it somewhat earlier than expected," she says, with a warm laugh. "But it was hard work, and this is only just the first step."

The reaction of others in the field to her new project varies: "Some think I'm completely mad, others think it's a good idea and very novel. We now have the difficult task of turning the idea into reality!"

Those who know Kearney will not be surprised by her unorthodox approach. Throughout her career she has championed patient-centred services and challenged traditional medical school thinking that views nursing as the poor relation to medicine – a point made recently in her lecture "Cancer nursing: gardeners

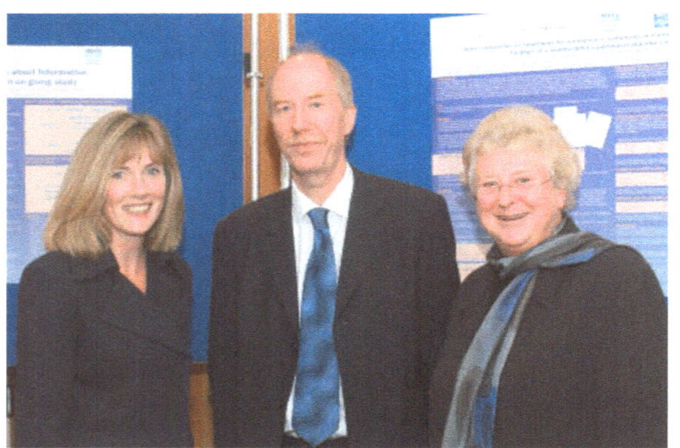

With Scottish Health Minister Malcolm Chisholm and Christine Hallett, Vice-Chancellor of Stirling University, at the opening of the Cancer Care Research Centre – Kearney's project from conception to completion

or people in the big house?". The title was prompted by hearing an eminent oncologist in Scotland use this particular metaphor to remind nurses of their "proper" role. "That is a prevailing attitude, unfortunately," she says. "I've had doctors say to me, 'Oh there is going to be money for nursing research, but none for basic cancer research,' to which I reply, 'This isn't about nursing, it is about patients.' Because I am a nurse, they have difficulty in disassociating that from what I'm trying to do."

Kearney is applauded by the European nursing community for her key role in increasing the resources and educational opportunities available to the 22,000 members of the European Oncology Nursing Society (EONS). As President of the Society (1997–99), she negotiated successfully with the leadership of the Federation of European Cancer Societies (FECS) for EONS (the only nurses' member of FECS) to be put on a more equal footing with the medical societies.

She has always championed patient-centred services and challenged traditional medical school thinking.

Last year, she was asked to present one of the nursing profession's most prestigious lectures, the Robert Tiffany Annual Nursing Lecture, which she delivered under the title: "Cancer nursing in the UK: Practice, policy... or just pretending?"

With characteristic courage, she "pulled no punches" in warning the audience that nurses were in danger of becoming sidetracked by battles over roles and titles. What did it matter, she argued, if it was a clinical nurse specialist or an advanced nurse specialist who delivered the best care to patients; what was more important was doing good research to find out what that best care is.

She received a standing ovation–unusual at professional conferences in the UK. "What was nice was the number of people who came up to me afterwards and said: That really made sense to me; it was about nursing and not about some academic thing."

Kearney says she is driven by a strong sense of wanting to do to something that makes a difference to patients. "It sounds twee, but that's why I became a nurse; that's why I do what I do; if I can make a difference at an individual patient level, then that is important. When I think things are unjust or unfair, then I am willing to put my head above the parapet and stand up for what I believe in."

This sometimes makes her unpopular with the policy makers she takes issue with through her presence on many national governmental and non-governmental committees.

But she also has her supporters. Gaining funding for the new patient-led research centre, for instance, will be helped, she believes, by the enlightened outlook of Scotland's current health minister, who she says has gone "outside the box" of the traditional thinking, based on a medical disease model, and recognises the need for healthcare services to be truly patient centred. "He is driving within Scotland at the moment a very direct push on patient involvement within health services."

Her style of communicating directly with the minister no doubt helped to speed things along, although it caused unrest in certain quarters. "My approach has always been: if you want something done, just speak to the person who is going to make the difference."

"When I think things are unjust or unfair, then I am willing to … stand up for what I believe in."

The Cancer Care Research Centre is an ambitious project, and Kearney is full of praise for her team, who she claims does most of the work. The first stage will be to engage with patients, carers and the general public at a very wide level to find out what their issues are concerning cancer and cancer care. "The plan is to go to mosques, synagogues, football grounds, bingo halls and supermarkets, and to put up stands saying: 'Come and tell us what you think about cancer and cancer care.'" This may sound somewhat evangelical, but Kearney believes it will be an effective way of reaching the 80% of patients who currently have no contact with existing support services or cancer support groups. The problems identified will inform changes to service delivery and raise research questions that the team will take forward.

Kearney describes herself as a "last minute person," who does not write "to do" lists or elaborate strategic plans, but "keeps it all in her head." She encourages her team, however, to work systematically to project plans, and is ready with guidance and motivational support when needed.

"When I go along to team meetings and say 'I've had another idea,' they say, 'Oh no!'–as they know they will have to implement it," she says with a smile.

She is clearly enthusiastic about being able to focus on research, after the administrative burden of her previous job as head of the School of Nursing and Midwifery at Glasgow University. The school was undergoing major change, and Kearney, then a senior lecturer, was offered the top position to improve research and education within the department.

"Suddenly I was responsible for everything, across the board: trying to manage a deficit, sorting out the department, trying to get our voice heard at faculty meetings, while keeping my cancer care research focus. It was hard juggling all these balls at once."

Under Kearney's leadership, student numbers went up and research income improved; though she is modest about her own part in turning things round. "A lot of it was about helping people regain confidence, and take responsibility themselves to move things forward."

"It was hard juggling all these balls at once."

At Glasgow she found it frustratingly hard to get a fair share of resources. "The Department of Nursing and Midwifery at the University of Stirling is much larger than at Glasgow, so we will be on a much more even footing with other academic disciplines," she says. "To invest in nursing on a significant scale, as they are doing, I think is very encouraging. It doesn't seem to be happening to the same extent in the more traditional universities."

Her research track record, which has yielded over 50 publications in peer-reviewed journals, bears testimony to the benefits of nursing interventions in improving the outcome for patients with cancer. "I'm not interested in doing academic esoteric research. What I want to do is work that is scientifically robust, and that is going to be useful clinically to patients."

Kearney's appointment at Stirling coincided with a personally difficult period of her life–her mother, Jean, was diagnosed with lung cancer. "It took six weeks to get her prescribed pain control medica-

tion. She had cognitive impairment and couldn't articulate her needs properly, but we, her family, could understand her. I can't understand why it took so long to sort out something as basic as pain control. It was really difficult as a daughter, being perceived as this professor of cancer care, and not being able to make things better."

Jean was cared for at home and in a nursing home until she was admitted to a hospice, where she died 10 days later–one year after the cancer was diagnosed. "We were told that the NHS had nothing to offer and that she would have to go into a private nursing home."

"I can't understand why it took so long to sort out something as basic as pain control."

This experience, she feels, highlights how hard it is for patients and carers to make themselves heard, and how far away we are yet from a fully patient-centred cancer care service. The fact that her mother had co-morbid conditions–atrial fibrillation, deep vein thrombosis and cognitive impairment–meant she did not fit into the disease-orientated model of healthcare. "That is outrageous: society has a growing elderly population, many of whom are going to have co-morbid conditions."

It is ironic that the problem of inadequate pain control should have affected Kearney so close to home: long before her mother's diagnosis, she had repeatedly raised the issue of why pain control is often so poor when proven methods of good control have been known for over 20 years. From her earliest days as a nurse, she would not rest until she

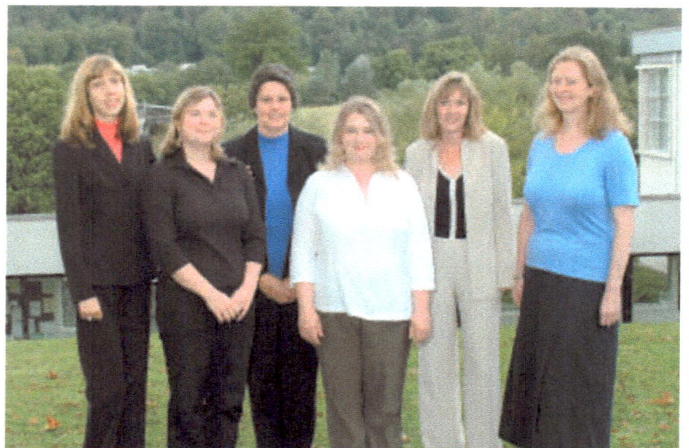

With her staff at the University of Stirling – recently voted the UK's most beautiful

had achieved optimal pain relief for her patients.

She is guided by principles of "pragmatic honesty" – being truthful, always doing the best you can – imparted by her parents as she grew up with her four sisters and two brothers in the small family home in the village of Milngavie (pronounced Mil-gie), seven miles north of Glasgow. It was a busy household, with uncles and aunts coming and going, and her mother was always ready to add a little extra something to the Sunday dinner pot to cater for whoever turned up.

It was at the age of three that she recalls first wanting to be a nurse "It was all I ever wanted to do." Her mum worked as an auxiliary nurse in a centre for disabled children, but this was when she was aged 10–long after her own desire to be a nurse emerged. Her father, Jack, worked first as a fireman and then as a docker in Glasgow.

She is guided by principles of "pragmatic honesty" – being truthful, always doing the best you can.

As the second youngest of seven children, she "had to have a degree of independence to survive." She was brought up in the Catholic faith, but recalls having a rebellious attitude against some of the doctrine. She also found it tiresome having to travel five miles to the nearest Catholic school, and if she had no key subjects, would stay away and work from home.

"My form teacher hauled me in because I hadn't been at school for a few days. He asked me what it was I wanted to do when I left school. I

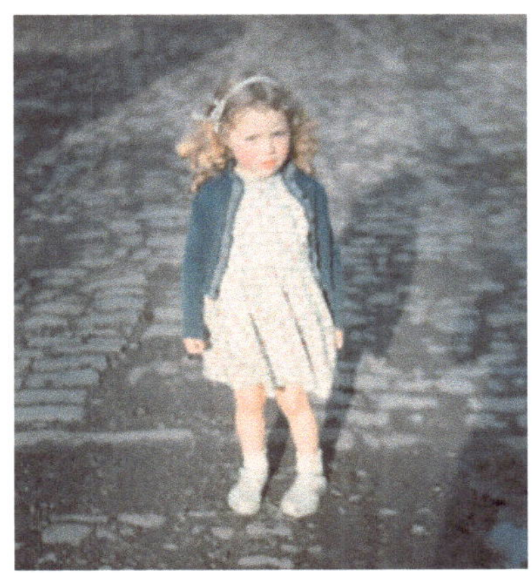

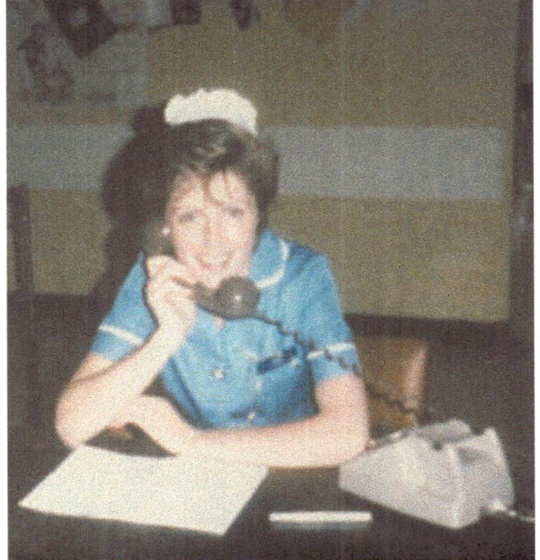

Setting out: From a very early age Kearney was determined to become a nurse. She qualified in 1981 and started her career in Glasgow.

told him I wanted to be a nurse and I had a place at Glasgow. He said: 'If I were lying in bed with two broken arms and two broken legs, and saw you coming up the ward, I would do my best to get out of your way – you are so irresponsible.' I've never forgotten it, and when I became a sister, I wanted to go back to him and say: 'See, you were wrong!'"

She qualified as a nurse in 1981 and worked for two years at Gartnavel General Hospital in Glasgow. It was a time of major life changes – she got married and had a son, Adam. And then a chance event, like so many career opportunities that occurred later, put her on the path to oncology nursing: having opted for a place on an acute medical ward, she found that half the ward had been allocated to oncology beds.

Faced with the demands of caring for acute medical patients with myocardial infarctions and the like, Kearney decided to do a course in intensive care. A job offer in intensive care followed, and she almost took that road. But fate intervened, again in favour of oncology. When she asked her boss for a reference for the intensive care job, she was offered promotion to ward sister, which she accepted. This led to a friendship with the ward's day-shift sister Phyllis Campbell (Kearney was then working nights), and they remain close friends some 20 years later. "Phyllis was the person who was always there for me. She has supported me through some difficult times–and stopped me doing mad things, like going off to become a lawyer midway through my career!"

"I wanted to go back to him and say: 'See, you were wrong!'"

Kearney's experience as an oncology ward sister enabled her to move to a new job as a clinical nurse specialist at the Beatson Oncology Centre in Glasgow. This led to a decision to boost her qualifications by doing a masters of science degree in clinical oncology at Glasgow University.

"It was unusual for a nurse to apply for the course, especially without having a first degree. It was the first year of the programme, and I went to see Stan Kaye and Anne Barrett, who were the professors in Glasgow at the time. They spoke to the medical faculty and were instrumental in

getting me a place. So it's their fault that I'm where I am today!"

Kearney was the only nurse on the course, along with seven medical registrars. She found the heavy science and physics modules "very tough," and she has strong memories of the pride she felt as her family attended her graduation in 1989.

In 1992, she left her job as clinical nurse specialist at the Beatson Oncology Centre to take up a teaching post as Macmillan Lecturer in Cancer Nursing at Glasgow University. After three years, she moved on to Edinburgh University to fulfil the same role there for a similar period. She then returned to Glasgow for a senior lecturer post, after which came a nine-month break from academia: she was seconded to the Commission for Health Improvement in London to manage an in-depth review of cancer services in England and Wales. "It was a wonderful opportunity to see healthcare from a different angle, and to link in with policy makers."

Kearney was the only nurse on the course, along with seven medical registrars.

While her experience working in London was valuable, there has been nothing career-wise down south to entice her away long-term from her beautiful homeland. Her Scottish nationality has helped to "open doors" in Europe, especially during her presidency of EONS.

"Scotland is a small country trying to make itself heard within a much larger administration; nurse leaders in countries such as Estonia can identify with that," she says.

Through EONS she made many good contacts and friends, including Anne Jaaksaar, head nurse of the Estonian Cancer Centre–"a wonderful committed person." Kearney obtained a grant from Brystol-Myers Squibb to go to Tallinn to help with the development of cancer nursing there. She recalls the desperate conditions, which were a legacy of the old Soviet rule. "Patients were crammed into small rooms with the tops and bottoms of the beds touching; there were no curtains, no privacy, no facilities and few drugs." A further grant allowed Jaaksaar to visit Scotland, which gave her a fresh perspective on cancer nursing. "Things in Tallinn have improved so much under her leadership."

A short time into her presidency of EONS, Kearney became aware of preliminary research aimed at sharing nursing information stored on patient records. She was quick to see the potential value of this work and how it could be practically realised through the involvement of the 22,000 nurse members of EONS. After a bout of energetic networking and negotiating, she arranged for EONS to provide the research network for the massive landmark WISECARE project, funded by a grant from the European Commission of almost 1 million ECUs. The acronym stands for Workflow Information Systems for European Nursing Care, and the project aims to improve cancer nursing practice and ultimately patient outcomes through the integration and use of state of the art information technology. EONS was one of five European partners in the WISECARE project, which involves 17 clinical sites in 10 European countries. Nurses enter information about patients' chemotherapy symptoms into a mini-electronic patient record. This automatically transforms the data into meaningful clinical information in the form of symptom scores and graphs.

"For the first time nurses across Europe were able to communicate with each other, learn from each other and share best practice," she says. The results of the first phase of the study demonstrated that a systematic approach to the assessment of patient symptoms improved patient outcome.

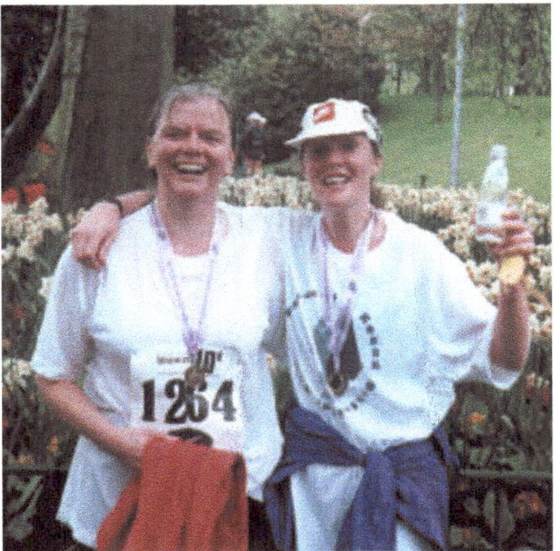

Running mates: with close friend Phyllis Campbell after the 1999 Glasgow Half Marathon

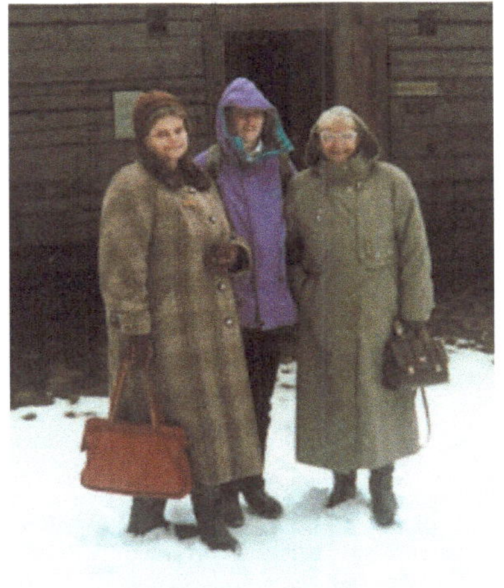

With nursing staff outside the Cancer Centre in Tallinn, Kearney spent time there in 1996, helping develop the Estonian cancer services

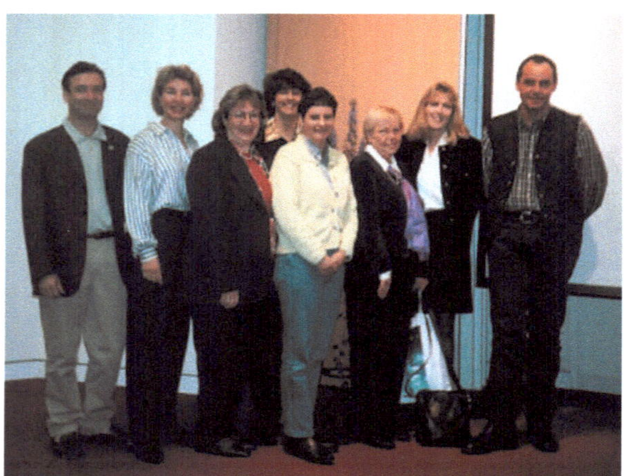

Members of the Board of the European Oncology Nursing Society, at the 1998 Spring convention in Leuven. Kearney's Presidency (1997–99) is remembered for her success in negotiating a more equal status for EONS with other groups in the Federation of European Cancer Societies

"The WISECARE project has had a profound effect on nursing care."

Nurses had seemed to be invisible within healthcare delivery; they found it difficult to articulate their worth within an increasingly cost-conscious healthcare system. Now they have hard evidence of the difference they make." It seems fitting that, as a gifted communicator, Kearney has been instrumental in revolutionising communication between nurses throughout Europe.

She remains principal investigator on the WISECARE project–now funded by the Royal Marsden Hospital–and has recently received a large grant from Vodafone Foundation UK to develop this work further, using mobile phone technology. The grant is funding a new study that aims to find out whether mobile phone technology used to moni-

tor symptoms in patients receiving chemotherapy for colorectal cancer can improve outcome. Patients will fill in their symptoms on mini-electronic patient records displayed on a phone screen. They will then press a button and the data will be uploaded in real time to a hospital-based system. If their symptoms are outwith certain control levels, a nurse will call them with appropriate advice.

"This is really quite exciting as this is the first time, as far as we are aware, that mobile phones have been used in symptom management in patients with cancer," she said. The new study is linked to the QUASAR 2 (Quick and Simple and Reliable) international study of bolus 5-fluorouracil/folinic acid versus capecitabine plus irinotecan as adjuvant treatment of colorectal cancer.

While Kearney sees modern technology offering great things for the sharing of good practice, she is concerned about one area that it cannot reach: the negative attitude of healthcare professionals to older patients with cancer. At the ECCO meeting in Copenhagen in October, she presented evidence from several studies which identified inadequacies in the care and treatment received by older patients with cancer compared with their younger counterparts. She has recently begun a major study of older people's perceptions of cancer information and treatment. Why is she such a strong advocate for better standards of care for older patients with cancer? "Because I became aware professionally and personally of the injustices in the care and treatment received by these patients."

Kearney deplores the paternalistic assumptions concerning older patients' wishes, made by health professionals "across the board" on the basis of their own value-laden attitudes. She calls for future research to identify the special needs of older people with cancer. "To do this, it must take account of the high frequency of co-morbid conditions, including cognitive limitations, and how these contribute to perceptions about cancer and its treatment. Older people with cancer are often treated as a single group; the reality is that they are individuals with different lifestyles, attitudes and coping strategies."

Asked what key quality marks her out, Kearney says determination. "I climbed Kilimanjaro earlier this year, and the only thing that got me to the top was determination." It was something she had long wanted to do, and when she saw an advert in the Guardian newspaper for a sponsored climb for the charity Voluntary Services Overseas, she jumped at it. Friends and family helped her raise the necessary £3,000 (54,300), and in February she flew off to Nairobi. From there it was an eight-hour bus journey to the Tanzanian basecamp. The four-day climb took the party through rain forest, moorland and alpine desert, before reaching the top where the temperature was –20°C.

Kearney was one of only five, out of the original party of 24, who reached Uhuru peak – the summit of Kilimanjaro, at around 19,300 feet (5,900 metres). Altitude problems, including raised intracranial pressure, forced the others to turn back. She herself had to cope with repeated bouts of vomiting. "It was nearly dawn as we approached the top and I was retching all over the place. I'm so glad I kept going. The views at the top were stunning – it was incredible."

Seeking out such life-changing experiences is in keeping with her philosophy of life, in which religion no longer plays a part. "I believe we

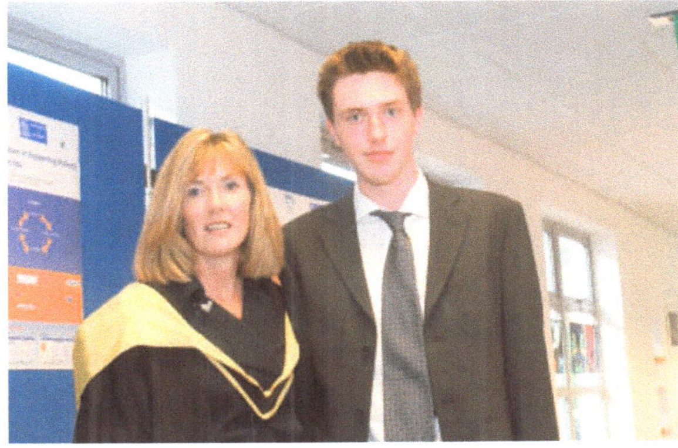

A Stirling relationship: son Adam studies philosophy at the same university

On her way to the summit of Mount Kilimanjaro. Determination is her defining characteristic, says Kearney

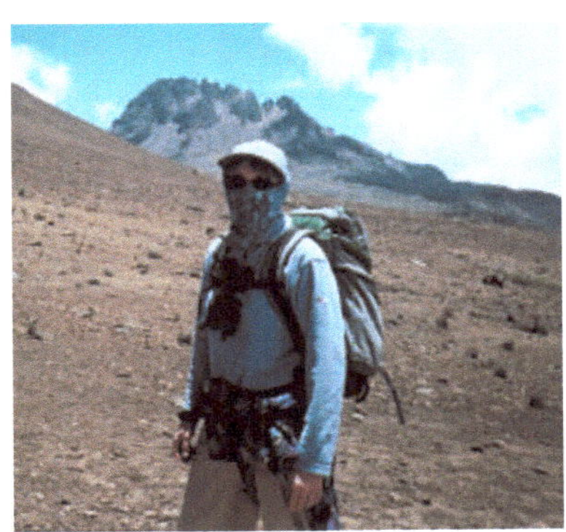

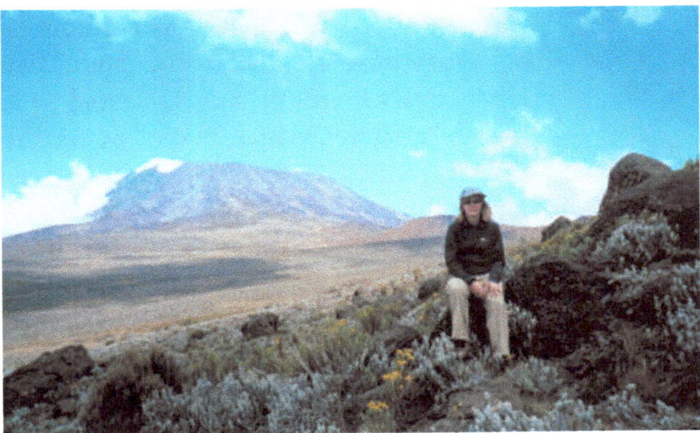

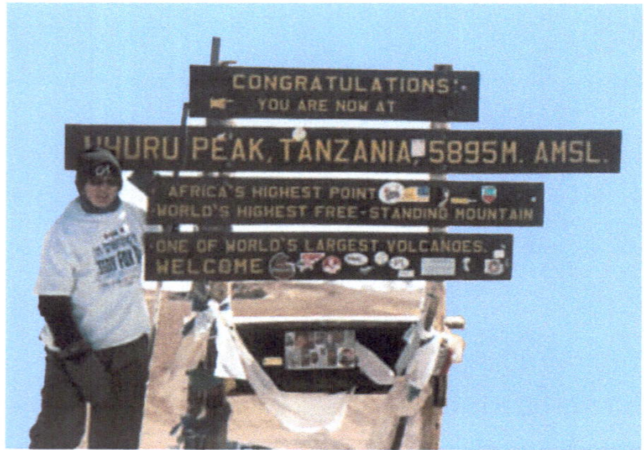

have one chance, and it is here and now; so you have to really go for it." Her main source of spiritual strength is through her friends, who "know my vulnerabilities and are very supportive."

She is very close to her son Adam, now 21, who happens also to be at Stirling University. "He was there first – doing his philosophy degree. We don't often bump into each other, as he is at the other end of the campus. But we meet at least once a month and I take him out and feed him."

Kearney unwinds at the weekend by hill-walking, and going to the gym three times a week helps keep her fit. She enjoys catching up on the Dickens classics she missed out on as a child, as well as contemporary novels – the last one being The Lovely Bones by Angela Sebold – "A beautifully written book." So far she has resisted the Russian literature Adam says she should read.

Her musical taste is wide – from Alice Cooper to Puccini, whose opera Madame Butterfly she has seen many times. Her favourite film is Wuthering Heights – the 1939 classic, with Lawrence Olivier playing Heathcliffe and Merle Oberon playing Cathy. "I've been married twice, in love once and remain a hopeless romantic."

But since taking on the professorship at Stirling, Kearney admits she has had little chance to get out to see a film or a play. "My friends are not happy I am working so hard," she says. She promises to try and do better next year. Though it looks set to be another busy one. Aside from the research commitments, she has work to complete on a comprehensive new textbook on cancer nursing; and her diary is filling up with governmental committee meetings and invited lecture dates.

She has exciting plans too for a holiday trip to Tuva, Outer Mongolia, with another friend, Alison Worth, who recently took up post as Senior Research Fellow at the Cancer Care Research Centre. Why Tuva? They had gone together to hear some Tuvan throat singers, which led her to read a book Tuva or Bust by Ralph Leighton. It tells the story of American physicist Richard Feynman's 10-year quest to travel to this distant exotic land of yaks, nomads and camels. Despite learning the language, and even the throat-singing technique, Soviet bureaucracy meant he died of cancer before he could fulfil his dream. "After reading the book I thought I must go there," says Kearney, who hopes they will be more successful than Feynman in reaching their destination. On arrival they will find the main mode of transport is on horseback. "Neither of us has ridden before," she says, "but that's not a problem; it's a minor detail!"

And one you can be sure that is not going to hold them back!

Paris and Helen Kosmidis:
A Legend in their Own Time

Jim McGuigan

When Paris Kosmidis, President of the European Medical Oncology Society, says that he intends to ensure that the European Union (EU) recognises medical oncology as a specialty throughout Europe within three to four years, you would do well to take him at his word.

For Kosmidis has a history. He can already claim much of the credit for the establishment of medical oncology in his home country Greece. While others may be content to celebrate their success in rising through the ranks, Kosmidis can reflect with pride on his role in building the very structures of the Greek medical oncology service, including the department he now heads at Hygeia Hospital in Athens.

Of course, the challenges are rather different this time round. Under Greek law, all it took to get medical oncology recognised as a specialty was to find 21 medical oncologists to form a professional society, which through increasing pressure convinced the government. If only the EU's legendary procedures could be that simple.

"There are several steps you must go through in order to gain official recognition of a profession (medical specialty) in Europe," says Kosmidis, sounding mildly exasperated. "First you have to gain approval from the relevant subcommittees, then the committees, then from the Parliament; and finally you need to go to the minister for health and the Prime Ministers – who only get together once a year at the summit meetings – to get the official signature. It takes years – the bureaucracy is unbelievable!"

Many countries in Europe still don't recognise medical oncology as an official specialty, and having seen what a difference it has made in his home country, Kosmidis is convinced that the prize is worth the fight. "Once we achieve this recognition, then each country will have an obligation to train young physicians in medical oncology and to organise hospitals so that patients receive better care."

With 10 new countries set to join the EU, Kosmidis knows his work

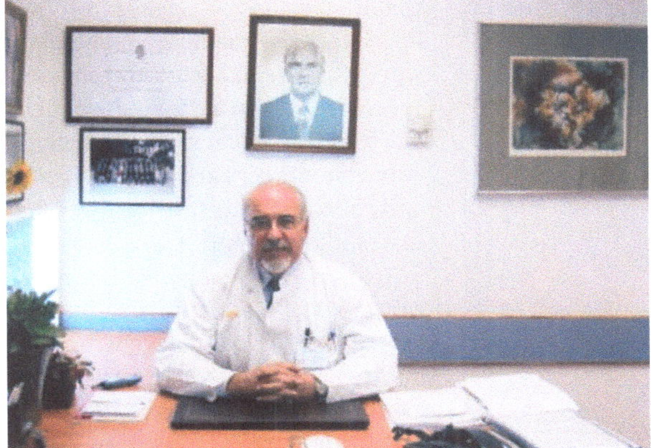

Paris Kosmidis in his office at Hygeia Hospital in Athens

is cut out, especially with regard to the lengthy lobbying that has to take place in Brussels, and along with others, he spends many hours talking to the members of European Parliament, to other societies and to patients' groups, at the national level and Europe-wide. But he recognises that it is not personal diplomacy alone that will swing it in the EU. The diverse parts of Europe's oncology community have spent many years gearing themselves up to maximise their voice within the increasingly powerful structures of the EU, and Kosmidis is counting on that paying off.

ESMO's influential National Representative Committee, which is made up of representatives of 33 European countries, is a critical force in the drive for Europe-wide recognition of medical oncology. "It's like a small 'Euro Parliament' – a network through which we communicate with each other; find out the problems in each country, and then give directions. I call it the back bone of ESMO," says Kosmidis, who chaired the committee for many years.

Another powerful ally is the Federation of European Cancer Societies, which carries tremendous weight because it speaks not just for Europe's medical oncologists, who could be expected to lobby for specialist status in their own field, but for all medical professionals involved in cancer care, from surgeons and paediatricians to oncology nurses, radiologists and researchers.

Getting EU recognition of medical oncology as a specialty is a top priority for Kosmidis, because it holds the key to so many other improvements. However, he has many other priorities for his Presidency of ESMO – for professionals and patients.

He is particularly conscious of the need to build up the next generation of medical oncologists, who will not only keep up the rate of new scientific discoveries in the treatment of cancer, but most importantly will ensure that the profession, as it is practised in clinics and hospitals throughout Europe, keeps up with the latest treatment methods.

"We are focused on young people aged 30 to early 40s, who have 25 years and more ahead of them to drive medical oncology forward." The first small group of young oncologists went through ESMO's Young Medical Oncologist Transitional Research Fellowship programme last year, spending three days at the internationally acclaimed Institut Gustav-Roussy in Paris. "The idea is to place them in a centre of excellence, to be trained in the latest techniques in molecular biology gene therapy and DNA cancerogenesis so that they can transfer these skills to other oncologists in their home countries. Many countries desperately need these skills. For example [the former] Yugoslavia has excellent young medical oncologists, but because so much of the country was destroyed, oncology training has plenty room for improvement." He has received "wonderful letters" of appreciation from last year's students and is busy making arrangements for the 2004 programme, which will take a group to the world-renowned Karolinska Institute in Stockholm.

"We focused on young peuple… who have 25 years and more ahead of them to drive medical oncology forward."

Improving the palliative care provided by medical oncologists is another important objective for Kosmidis, who is saddened by recent evidence showing that some oncologists still do not see palliative care or the comforting of a deeply depressed patient as part of their job. Asked whether a cancer physician is the best placed for this role, he says, "It is a team job, but the physician is the team leader. Just a few minutes holding a patient's hand, not just as a doctor but as an equal, really showing they care, makes such a difference. Then he can explain that his colleague the team psychologist will come and talk further with the patient."

This brings the conversation round to another of Kosmidis' priorities: getting the medical oncology community to recognise patients as equal partners with their physicians. Here he can expect at least the level of resistance from the profession that is still being mounted against taking responsibility for palliative care and the wider well-being of the patient. Accepting an equal partnership with patients means that physicians not only have to provide the best treatment, but they have to explain to the patient about their disease and their treatment, they have to engage with the patient's views, and be prepared to face critical questions over the treatment options they are recommending. It is a major cultural change in what has traditionally been a very paternalistic occupation. And many in the profession see it as a serious threat. Not so Kosmidis, who has been pushing ahead with putting his ideas on equality into practice by opening up the last ESMO congress with president Dr Heinz Ludwig to some 200 patients, many of whom were given travel expenses to attend special presentations put on specifically for patients and their families.

"Just a few minutes holding a patient's hand makes such a difference."

At this year's congress in Vienna, he wants to go a step further by al-

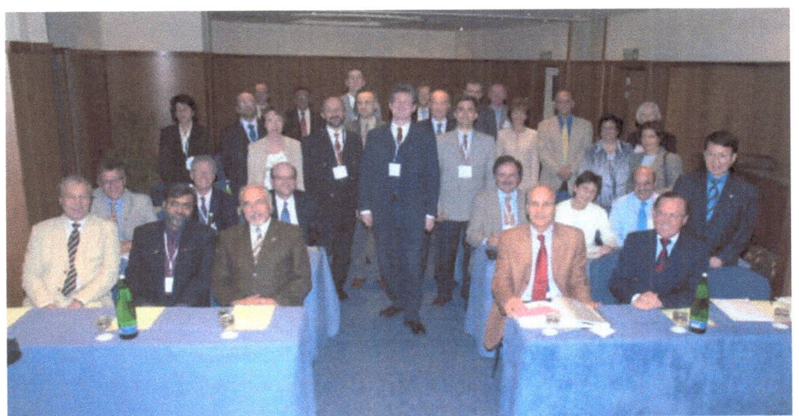

The National Representative Committee of ESMO. Kosmidis, seated at the right of the table on the left, chaired this influential body for many years

lowing patients to attend the specific scientific sessions, if it is not prohibited by the law. Is he not concerned that sessions could be "hijacked" by patients putting over their own personal agenda? "The sessions are chaired by people trained in guiding people away from personal details to the broader picture, and most patients will go along with this approach," he says. "I think anything that helps the communication between doctors and patients regarding, for example, treatment options is mutually beneficial."

Kosmidis' preference for forging his own path rather than following in the footsteps of others showed itself from an early age. The choice of pursuing a career in medicine was his alone, and had no precedent anywhere else in his family. His grandparents on both his mother's and his father's side had fled their homes in Constantinople (now Istanbul) to escape the war between Greece and Turkey in 1922, leaving everything behind them. They arrived in Athens with nothing more than the clothes they stood up in: "They had lost everything they had owned there, and came to Athens starting from zero – or five below zero." His father, Thanos, had been six years old at the time; his mother was actually born on board the ship that took her family to safety.

He wants to go a step further by allowing patients to attend the specific scientific sessions…

Paris was born just after the end of the Second World War. "It was a time of post-war austerity, in which my father, mother, and brother all shared the same room; I remember it well," he says. Despite the shortage of material comforts, Kosmidis remembers it was a very happy household.

His father built up a successful business importing wool and manufacturing blankets with it, and he would have liked Paris to follow him into the family business, as his younger son had done. But Paris had other plans. He enrolled at Athens University as the first member of his family to study medicine. Why medicine? "I don't know. I used to spend many hours visiting my father in hospital. He suffered from Addison's Disease. That may have been a factor."

The Addison's disease eventually led to his father suffering a fatal myocardial infarction, but not before he saw Paris qualify in his chosen profession. "I think he was very proud. He died in my arms in 1984. My brother took on the family business and has continued its success."

In 1969, to complete his in-service training as a doctor, Kosmidis wanted to go to the US. Greece was under a military dictatorship at this time, and, first, he had to complete his national military service, in the navy, followed by one year of Obligatory Rural Area Service. He chose the island of Crete, and he fondly recalls the simple kindness and gratitude of the local farmers who presented him with everyday problems, ulcers, asthma, stroke and the usual ailments. He knew, however, that he was not cut out for that sort of work: "I could never have become a general practitioner," he says, "I wanted more detailed scientific knowledge of each disease."

It was during his last few months on Crete, in 1972, that a young physician, Helen Vasilatou, arrived on the island to do her Obligatory Rural Area Service. "She was very intelligent, and I admired her because she treated her patients so carefully and with love," he recalls.

The two young doctors helped each other in different ways; he passed on what he had learned in the hospital over the previous nine months and he was grateful to be updated on new techniques he had missed out on during his three years in national military service. "I remember her planning the treatment of a patient; she put in a few things, different approaches that I could learn from."

Their work together blossomed into romance, and when he left Crete a few months before Helen, they were already engaged and planning a life together. Kosmidis flew off to the US in 1973 and completed his training at Sinai Hospital in Detroit. He then served as a Fellow in haematology – oncology at two other Detroit hospitals: Wayne State University and Henry Ford Hospital. He returned to Greece to marry Helen – a big Greek wedding – and then they both travelled out to Detroit, where Helen also gained a hospital appointment.

Working in oncology in the US was a revelation for the young Kosmidis. "For the first time I saw patients with cancer being treated." This was not something he had ever considered possible, as the attitude in Greece at that time, as in many other countries where oncology remained undeveloped, was: "It's cancer. There is little that can be done."

"I was astonished when I saw patients with cancer being treated very effectively all of the time and well supported most of the time; after

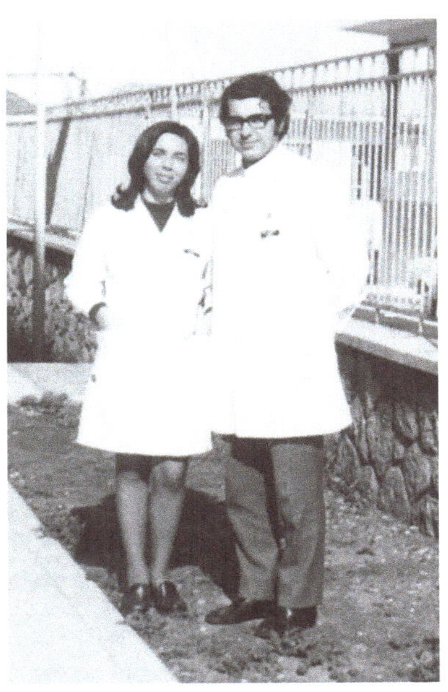

this, there was no other subject for me but oncology."

His research interests soon centred on combining different therapies in lung cancer, to see which regimen was the best; predominant among these were the taxanes, which at that time were just emerging as powerful new agents.

Working in oncology in the US was a revelation for the young Kosmidis. "For the first time I saw patients with cancer being treated."

The pull of Greece was strong, however, and in 1979 he returned home, determined to get medical oncology officially recognised as a specialty and properly established in Greece. He found that another Athens physician, Dr George Stathopoulus, shared his vision, and together they sought out more like-minded physicians in order to gather the 21

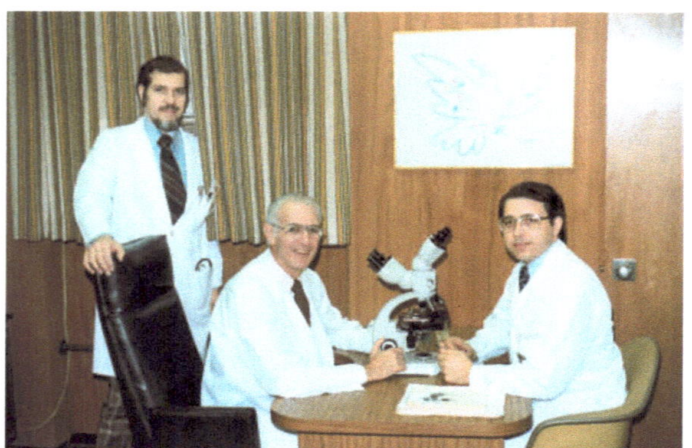

With Professor Arnold Axelrod (centre) and Dr Chris Palacas, at Wayne State University, Michigan, where Kosmidis served as Fellow in haematology-oncology after completing his training

needed under Greek law to set up a professional society. They did this, and in 1980 set up the Hellenic Medical Oncology Society. Kosmidis then set about developing a network of good research centres. Together with Dr George Fountzilas and another two colleagues, they founded the Hellenic Cooperative Oncology Group, which rapidly took off. The

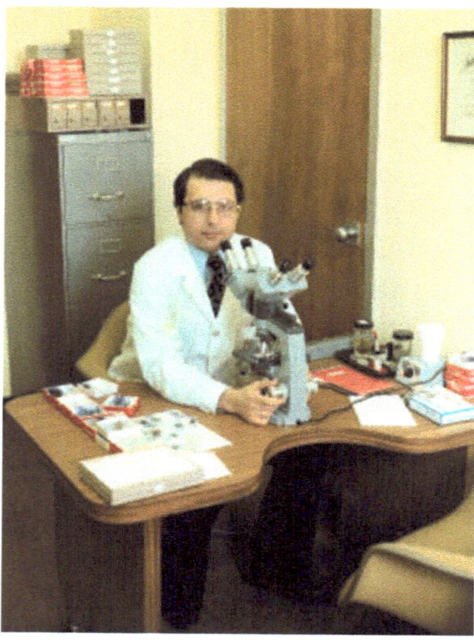

On the job

four centres it started off with have now increased to 25.

"This was a very important stage in my career. Once we had set up the research network everything else followed, support from industry, recruiting people, buying computers, hiring statisticians and starting to publish papers."

Kosmidis clearly loves the scientific quest involved in medical research. "One of the things I enjoy most is when I'm at the computer with the statistician, with all the data printing out. It's like the last minute of a sports game–when you are waiting for the final result. You look to see the shape of the curve, to see if it is going to be above or below that of the placebo."

One of his papers from the Hellenic Cooperative Oncology Group to make an international impact was a series of studies, published in the Journal of Clinical Oncology and in Annals of Oncology, on the use of taxanes to treat patients with lung cancer. "We found the treatment had improved the quality of life of the patient and prolonged it." These quality research papers along with many others from other colleagues helped raise Greece's standing in the international league of medical oncology research publications from nowhere to a place among the top ten.

Once we had set up the research network everything else followed.

Keen to build on this success, Kosmidis proposed holding the 1998 ESMO Congress in Athens. Having put medical oncology firmly on the map in his own country, and raised

the specialty's research profile internationally, he had a strong case. The
venue was agreed, and he spent three
years organising the meeting, which
attracted 6,000 delegates and was a
great success for medical oncology
in Greece, and for him personally.
He soon began to find himself dealing more and more with international matters.

This chain of successes culmi-
nating in the high profile 23rd ESMO
congress helps to explain how a
young man from a non-medical family on the margins of Europe managed to attain what is considered to
be the most prestigious position in
European medical oncology.

In 2001, the Hellenic Cooperative Oncology Group's achievements
were recognised by his country who
honoured the founders with the
Award of the Academy of Athens. "It
was one of the proudest moments in
my life," he says.

One might imagine that even
Greece, which has given so much
to world medicine, would only have
room for one Kosmidis. But one
would be wrong, for Paris Kosmidis
is in reality part of a great oncology
double act. His partner, Helen Kosmidis ("Dr Vasilatou" according to
her father – she took the Kosmidis
name when she married, because
her American colleagues found it
easier to pronounce!) has played an
equally important role as one of the
founding mothers of Greek paediatric oncology.

Like Paris, Helen, who grew up
on the island of Cephalonia – made
famous by the novel Captain Corel-
li's Mandolin – was the first in her
family to study medicine. And she
too studied at Athens University and
qualified with flying colours, though

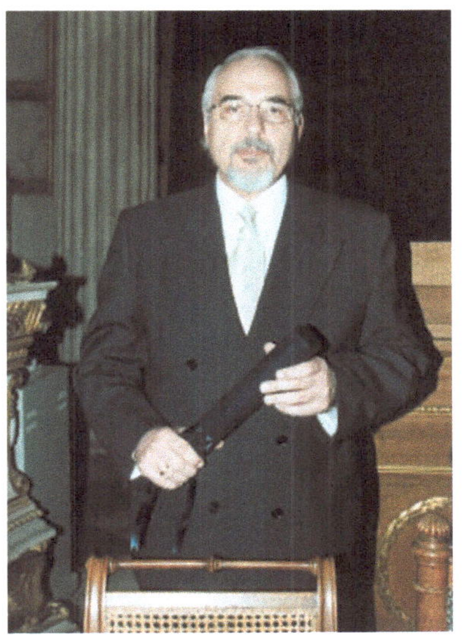

After receiving
the Award of the
Academy of Athens
2001, "It was one
of the proudest
moments of my
life"

it was not until they were both sta-
tioned in Crete for their Obligatory
Rural Area Service that they actually met. The period spent working
in Detroit after their marriage was a
revelation to both of them, and the
determination to bring home the
best parts of the oncology care they
had experienced in the US burned
as brightly in Helen as it did in her
husband.

Paris Kosmidis is in reality part of a great oncology double act.

That determination led to her
founding, along with other colleagues, the Hellenic Paediatric
Oncology Society, which has now
revolutionised the quality of care
of children with cancer throughout
Greece. In Helen's case, however,
the term "mother" of Greek paediatric oncology means much more
than this; it can be taken almost literally. For Helen's commitment is
a very personal one, and she refers
to all her patients as her "children."

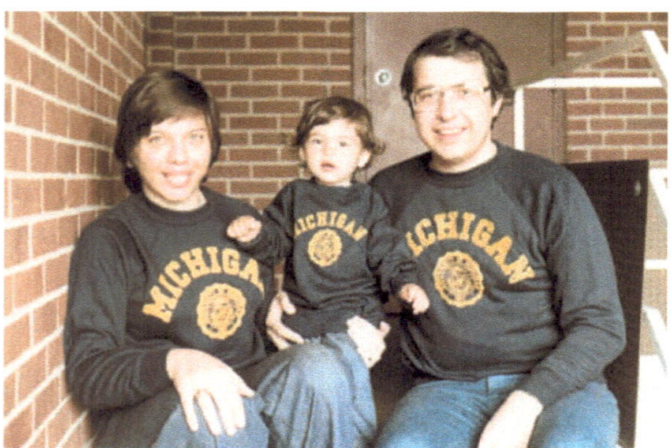

Paris and Helen with daughter Sofia aged 2

As her daughter once explained to a visiting relative: "Mother has lots of children but only three of them live here."

One of the most rewarding aspects of her work, she says, is the strong bond she develops with the children as they grow. "I don't call them survivors, but winners," she says. Understandably, she also enjoys strong ties with the parents, who must think the world of her. "I get a card at Christmas or a call to ask how I am doing, not just from parents whose children pulled through, but from the others too. This means so much to me."

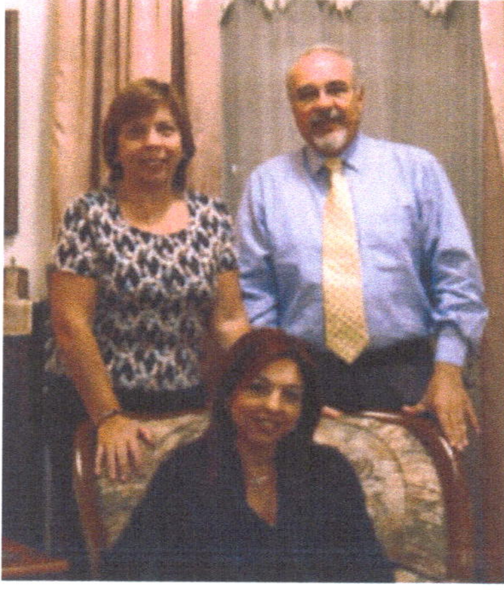

The same family group many years on. Sofia now has an oncology career of her own

Helen is also very active on the research side, with a particular interest in the psychosocial aspects of cancer care of young people – a subject on which she has written a number of papers, published in Medical Paediatric Oncology and other peer-reviewed journals. Another of Helen's aspirations is to convince people that adolescent oncology can be covered by paediatrics. Adolescents are a distinct group of patients with many needs, and they have paediatric-type malignancies in three out of four of cases.

As her daughter once explained: "Mother has lots of children but only three of them live here."

This oncologist partnership between Helen and Paris that has done so much for cancer care in Greece may seem an obvious one with hindsight. Yet when they first met, in Crete, marrying a doctor was not what this highly competent newly qualified female medic had in mind. "The ones I had met thought that all women doctors should be in the lab doing microbiology!" she laughs.

But Paris, it seems, was different, and won her heart. They married, and were immediately faced with the inevitable decision about where the two of them would pursue their independent careers. With her excellent French language skills, Helen had her heart set on Paris – the city that is. But Detroit won in the end, "because Paris said it would be easier for me to improve my English than for him to learn French."

The return to Greece in 1979, however, was a move that suited them both, and allows each of them to work in their separate fields to

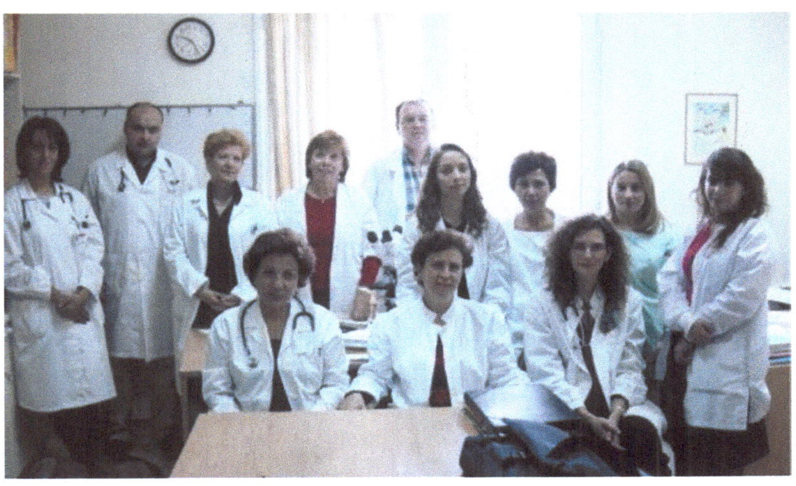

their full potential, and to stunning effect. They are both devoted to their work, and the hour spent each day over breakfast, and again over a late supper, are often the only time they really have to themselves. Do they ever sound each other out on particular cases? "Not really, but we do share problems, and help each other to look at things in different ways."

"The ones I had met thought that all women doctors should be in the lab doing microbiology!"

The couple have three children. Sofia, the eldest has followed her parents into oncology, though she has found her own space as a radiation oncologist trainee in Athens. Being a "Kosmidis" in the Greek cancer scene obviously carries a certain legacy, but they are all determined to ensure Sofia is able to be her own person and find her own career pathway. Their eldest son Thanos, aged 24, is working in the US in information technology, for a company that was instrumental in creating the Internet. Spyros, aged 19, is studying political sciences at Athens University, "We have great discussions about all the issues of the day."

They try to leave weekends free for the family, who all get together for lunch–apart from Thanos, who they often call so they can at least talk together.

Helen is careful to preserve a life outside of her work. She greatly enjoys music and, as an accomplished pianist, enlivens many family celebrations with her renditions of classical and popular music. Another love of her busy life is reading, and she recommends Middlesex by Pulitzer Prize-winning author Jeffrey Eugenides. This mesmerising saga of a near-mythic Greek American family and the roller-coaster ride of a single gene through time has special significance for her, being set mainly in Detroit.

Paris claims he has little time for non-medical reading, even his weekends are taken up with working on the several book chapters or draft lectures he always has under-

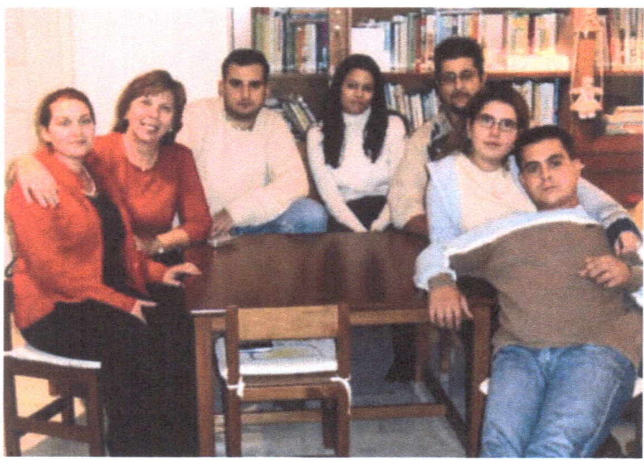

way. However, he finds he has got a lot out of reading about the exodus of Greek people from Turkey during the war of 1922. "I am fascinated to learn how these people coped with this pressure; it is the story of my family and maybe I am trying to understand myself more."

Listening to Greek music is one of the pastimes he most enjoys, his favourite composer being Mikis Theodorakis – best known outside of Greece for composing Zorba the Greek, the film score for the Third Man. "He was a communist and was put in prison just after the Second World War. Some of his best work was written in prison and listening to it, feeling the strength of the instruments, you gain insight into his interior world."

On religious matters, he is liberal in his Greek Orthodox faith, and he admits to being vexed by how so much inhumanity can occur under the eyes of God. But no doubts are put over to his patients. "I encourage patients to use their faith, because whatever gives them power will help them."

Helen too is careful to respect the religious beliefs of the families she is involved with. The vulnerability of human life is a reality that she lives with as part of her daily working life. "I can't believe that everything stops at death. I believe that if I die my spirit is going to be here, protecting my children," she says, referring of course to her large family of young patients, "but I still have things to do here."

Her next challenge is to get more radiotherapy equipment for the paediatric oncology service, which is currently being run down on the grounds that fewer children need it–a move Helen feels could deny some patients the treatment they need. "There are still a number of children who need radiotherapy for curative treatment or for palliation," she says.

"I believe that if I die my spirit is going to be here, protecting my children."

Paris, meanwhile, is looking forward in January to the results of his latest study comparing single-agent gemcitabine therapy with a combination of gemcitabine and carboplatin. "If it works, thousands of people will benefit from the lower side effect profile and increased convenience of taking one drug instead of two."

In four years he will be 60 and there seems so much to do. My only regret is that I didn't start earlier. "I think I could do more if I had more time–with the experience I have received now. I hope with the experience I gain at ESMO, I will be useful later toward some other aspect of European oncology or world oncology."

Helen and Paris. The historic significance of this partnership is

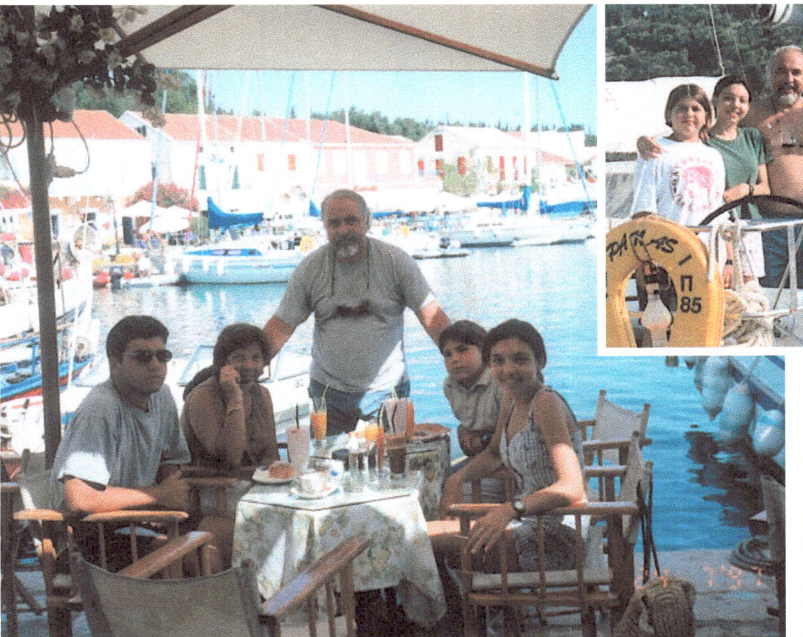

The Kosmidis
family enjoying
drinks together on
the harbour front,
and (inset) on
holiday in
Cephalonia

not lost on the Greek population, for whom the legend of Paris's love for beautiful Helen of Troy, and the terrible toll of death and destruction that followed in its wake, forms part of the country's identity.

It's as if their modern namesakes, who have earned their own place in the history of Greek medicine, have come back to redeem the Helen and Paris legacy. Their love for one another this time round bringing to Greece nothing but caring and healing.

"We both love what we are doing, we love each other, and we love family life," says Helen. "It is very important for a person to be happy in their job or life. I think if I was to be born again, I would do the same things again."

Jacek Jassem: Reaching out From Gdansk

MARC BEISHON

The success of the Fourth European Breast Cancer Conference – the world's second largest breast cancer event – will owe much to the dynamism of its chair this year, Jacek Jassem. He very actively supported his colleagues Martine Piccart and Louis Mauriac in persuading the EORTC (European Organisation for Research and Treatment of Cancer) to accept a proposal from the European Society of Mastology (EUSOMA), at that time led by Umberto Veronesi, to jointly organise a European conference on breast cancer that also included the breast cancer advocacy movement Europa Donna. Yet, few in the audience will be aware of Jassem's deep commitment to fostering international cooperation. His background as a young, idealistic cancer practitioner in communist Poland is the clue – and it has fuelled a seemingly inexhaustible reservoir of energy that propels Jassem around the world, before returning unerringly to his beloved home base of Gdansk in northern Poland.

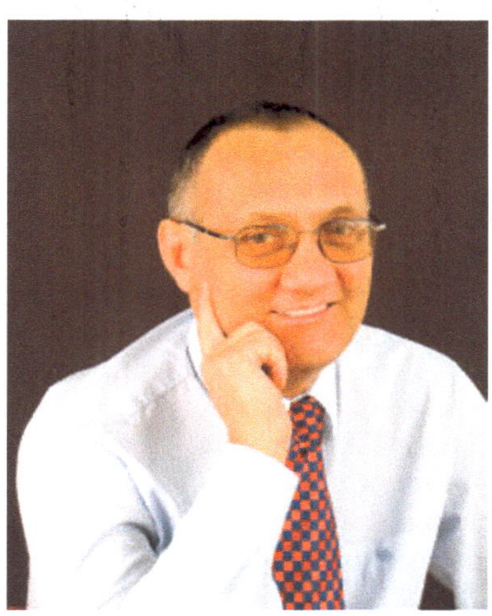

"Some people in the EORTC breast cancer group were not that enthusiastic at first about extending the conference to involve partners that are not strictly research bodies," says Jassem. "But it has proved to be a good decision. Instead of diluting the scientific content – as some had feared – we have been able to attract more good speakers to this much larger conference, and in my opinion the science input is now much higher than in the past."

As he adds, the critical mass obtained by combining the conferences of the EORTC, EUSOMA and Europa Donna has also raised the bar as far as media interest is concerned. "We can 'sell' much more to the media with our format of debates, symposia, teaching lectures and interaction with the audience with voting systems," he says. Sessions for lay people and patient management workshops add to a mix he feels is maximising potential to raise the profile of all the options for treating and caring for breast cancer sufferers – and, as will become apparent,

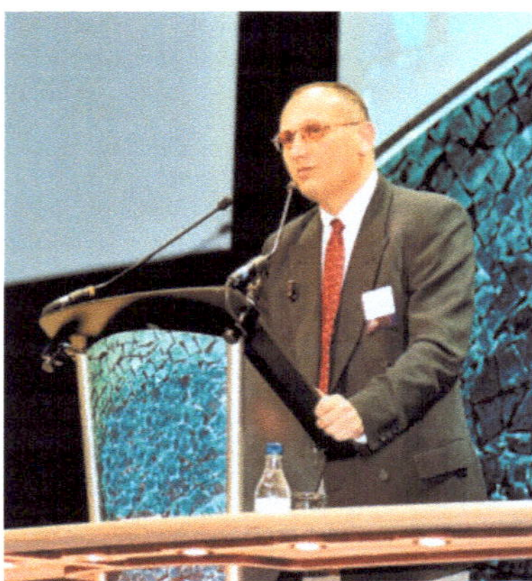

At the
microphone

Jassem is no inward facing physician.

Jassem's "day job" is head and professor of the Department of Oncology and Radiotherapy at the Medical University of Gdansk. He is also the chief oncology consultant for northern Poland, and senior administrator of cancer research in the country. On top of all this, he chairs the Central and East European Oncology Group, and is past and present chair and member of many other organisations, including the EORTC breast cancer group, but life revolves around the hospital in Gdansk.

In the grounds of the Medical University of Gdansk, where Jassem heads the Department of Oncology and Radiotherapy

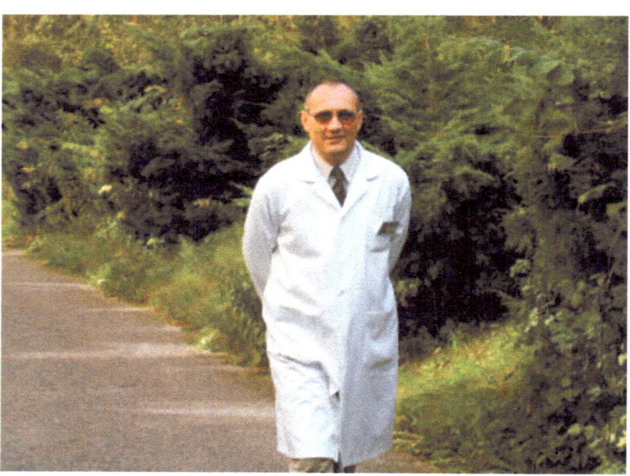

He explains: "I run a very busy department – we are one of two centres for cancer therapy in this part of Poland and we also teach medical students." Radiotherapy is carried out virtually round the clock, and the department caters for some 2,000 new patients a year – not counting those treated with other methods.

Unlike other large Polish cities, Gdansk, which together with its surrounding towns has a population of more than two million, has no dedicated cancer centre. It is Jassem's ambition to set one up, but conditions aren't easy.

"We are still in a difficult phase of development economically in Poland – we suffer from shortages of resources, so the only realistic option is to establish the new centre as a private unit. We have interest from industry abroad – but Poland's insurance system is also in transition, and private investors are very cautious about how they will get their money back. And in any case we have no tradition of private hospitals in Poland."

"Private investors are very cautious about how they will get their money back."

Poland, of course, is one of the countries set to become a full member of the European Union (EU) this year. It is a step that Jassem warmly welcomes, but he recognises that the country's tough economic circumstances will not change overnight. Indeed, like his approach to oncology, he sees progress as being by small but significant stages, rather than major breakthroughs. Yet if it hadn't been for one major upheaval, his career would have taken a very different path.

That event was the collapse of communism in Poland in 1989, which occurred shortly after Jassem had "escaped" to take up a fellowship at the Netherlands Cancer Institute in Amsterdam. Had it not been for the possibilities thrown up by the end of the old regime, Jassem's departure from his homeland – as with many of his fellow Poles – could have become permanent.

Jassem was born in Cracow in 1951, with the twin fortunes of having parents who were both academics – university professors in fact – and growing up in a city that largely escaped the destruction visited on other Polish cities during the Second World War. "Cracow is Poland's most beautiful city – I have very good memories of a wonderful tradition with very special people," says Jassem. He says his father survived the Warsaw Uprising during the war, where 100,000 young people – "a lost generation" – were killed. Both his parents went on to become professors of biology, and he also had a highly academic uncle – a famous Polish professor of phonetics.

"It was expected I would go to university too, but I only decided on medicine at a late stage, as I planned to study human sciences at first," says Jassem. Like many cancer specialists, it was the challenge of both medicine and then oncology that drove him on his present course. "Medicine is always a personal challenge no matter what you do, and when I finished my studies I looked for yet more challenge in oncology. I graduated in 1975 – at that time, oncology was even more of a challenge

than now – we had many more failures than successes. But in 30 years you can see huge progress."

Jassem did all his medical training in Gdansk, starting out in 1969 in a city he describes as "fantastic, with a long and rich history. We celebrated its millennium recently," with a mix of peoples, and a strong Dutch architectural influence. "Many important events took place here, such as the beginning of the Second World War and the start of the Solidarity union." Jassem's support for Solidarity and the anti-communism movement was to land him in trouble and stymie his progress for a long period.

"At that time, oncology was even more of a challenge than now."

His first research interest in oncology was on melanoma, "a fashionable topic then," and he duly completed a PhD, "Immunotherapy of malignant melanoma with BCG," in 1980. He spent a lot of time in the immunology lab – working mainly at night, as his main work was as a clinician.

Then Jassem moved to one of his two primary subjects, lung cancer (breast cancer of course being the other). "The incidence of lung cancer in Poland was growing very rapidly, and we were asked by the government to coordinate a nationwide research programme dealing mainly with the clinical aspects of the disease. Jassem's head of department, professor Tadeusz Zielinski, died shortly after this work was allocated, and he and a colleague then carried it on for the next five years or so.

"This was very efficient work – we coordinated the first large inter-institutional studies in Poland. We also developed a structure for other clinical trials in the country and increased the level of patient care, and the outcome was evident in a number of papers published in high-ranking journals."

Jassem's work with lung cancer led to him to helping set up the Central European Lung Cancer Conference, which convenes for the ninth time this September, when it will be held for the second time in Gdansk with, inevitably, Jassem as chairman. "This is the only pan-European lung cancer conference with a long tradition," he says. "We are expecting about 700 people, not just from Europe but from America, Japan and other countries. It's a large conference and a major global event in lung cancer this year."

"We coordinated the first large inter-institutional studies in Poland."

Research on lung cancer is one of the main interests of Jassem and his team at the Medical University at present, in particular molecular biology studies. "We have a very efficient multidisciplinary team here," he says, noting that the department also has one of the largest frozen lung tissue banks in Europe. "We've been approached for a large project recently from the Netherlands, because we can offer many more cases from our tumour bank," he says.

Polish rules on gathering material for translational research are another advantage Jassem and his colleagues have on their side. Unlike the more restrictive EU regulations, Polish rules currently allow the use of tissue for future research purposes. This is an option they risk losing on Poland's accession to the EU, and Jassem is adamant about the need to convince the European Parliament that the even tighter EU consent procedure, the Clinical Trials Directive due to come into force this May, could stop "absolutely essential" translational research.

Jassem has already had plenty of experience working under constraints, and he became increasingly frustrated by the stifling of scientific progress through lack of resources and international contacts during the communist era. Members of his family, he says, were soldiers in the home army (Armia Krajowa) during the war, and after the war ended never accepted the communist system.

After the government started clamping down on anti-Soviet activities, Jassem remembers in 1968, "many university people, mainly of Jewish origin, were kicked out of their positions. It was a big shock for me as a young man. Even before, I was critical of the political situ-

"We coordinated the first large inter-institutional studies in Poland."

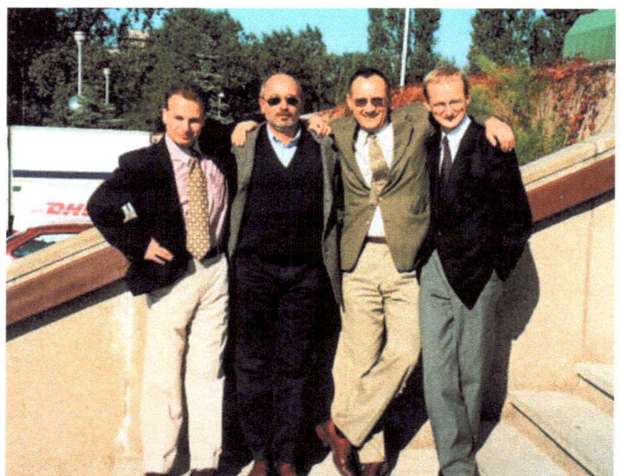

ation, but it was a turning point in my attitude. Starting then, I was very strongly against the system."

His desire to help the country break free of the Iron Curtain led Jassem to become active in the anti-communist movement and to support Lech Walesa's Solidarity movement. He was a witness to demonstrations in Gdansk, even attending – with difficulty – to injuries suffered by protesters. Eventually, in 1982, he was detained by the authorities in prison, but thankfully was let out after a few days, after a university official intervened on his behalf. Other colleagues were not so fortunate, and indeed Jassem's own brother, Piotr, spent six months in detention in the early 1980s, before being offered the chance to emigrate to Canada, where he still lives today.

Jassem had already worked abroad, having landed a student job in the endocrine lab at the Karolinska Hospital in Stockholm, and he subsequently made a research visit to the famous "Radiumhemmet" (Department of Radiotherapy). "This journey was covered from the money I had earlier earned in the same hospital. It was the late professor Jerzy Einhorn, then director of the Radiumhemmet – and founder of modern Swedish oncology – who made this visit possible."

**He was a witness
to demonstrations in Gdansk,
even attending
– with difficulty – to injuries.**

But further attempts to foster international contacts met with the usual obstacles, such as weeks spent waiting for visas, and lack of money to travel. As he recalls, when he first

set out to cooperate with EORTC – he was later to become chair of its breast group among other roles – he eventually arrived in the West with no money, even to buy meals. As he says: "I was supposed to attend meetings abroad twice a year – but it was difficult if each time I had to spend a whole day just queuing for a visa."

"But I got a lot of support – and credit – from people in EORTC, and after a few years we were able to prove we were a good partner. I am very proud of the fact that I was pioneer of this type of cooperation in Poland." Jassem mentions professor Joop van Dongen from the Netherlands Cancer Institute as being particularly helpful in extending the invitation to join the EORTC breast cancer group. "He took the risk with us as the first institute from eastern Europe."

Jassem's first training as an oncologist was in radiotherapy – but later he went on to carry out work in medical oncology as well. As he points out: "When I did radiotherapy, there was no such speciality in Poland as medical oncology, and I

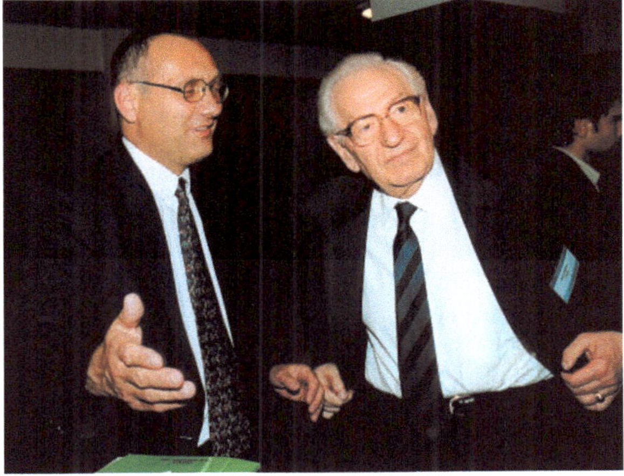

never considered it important to do a formal specialisation in the subject. Later, though, I realised I had to take a formal examination and it was great fun for the board here to have a professor up before them.

"People abroad ask me how it's possible to do both radiotherapy and medical oncology – I say I do my best. But breast cancer is an example where the two modalities are used in the majority of patients – it's more difficult if you have one specialist to irradiate the breast and another to administer chemo- or endocrine therapy. Here we can do both in one place and it is very beneficial."

In any case, adds Jassem, one of his main interests is the combination of radiotherapy and chemotherapy – "I've written a number of articles and book chapters, such as in the Oxford Textbook of Oncology."

"People abroad ask me how it's possible to do both radiotherapy and medical oncology – I say I do my best."

Jassem did indeed achieve his goal of becoming a full professor at the Department of Oncology and Radiotherapy – with dual specialities

under his belt – but that was only after he thought he'd probably left Poland for good. During the 1980s, his anti-establishment practices meant that he was overlooked for promotion to head the department, and indeed it ran without a head for eight years or so.

The rector of the university – a member of the communist party – and other university officials were so suspicious of Jassem that it was considered too risky for him even to address students at a summer scientific camp. "By that time I was so involved with international studies that when I was offered a one-year fellowship in the Netherlands I decided to go."

He was invited to the Netherlands Cancer Institute by professor Harry Bartelink, "one of my biggest mentors. I spent a fabulous year in the Netherlands with my family – and everyone in Gdansk was pretty sure this was my last journey to the West. It was a common solution then – many decided to leave Poland."

Jassem was then offered the chance to head the Department of Radiotherapy at one of the Dutch universities: "It was a very challenging proposal and I had talks with the dean and faculty, but we then had the first free election in Poland and the communist system collapsed. So I had a big dilemma: a chance to change my life, earn good money and enjoy new scientific possibilities in the Netherlands, or return to Poland. But I decided I had to go back – the bigger challenge was to see how the new situation in Poland would change my possibilities there."

His wife Ewa, who now heads the Department of Allergology at the Medical University, and daughters

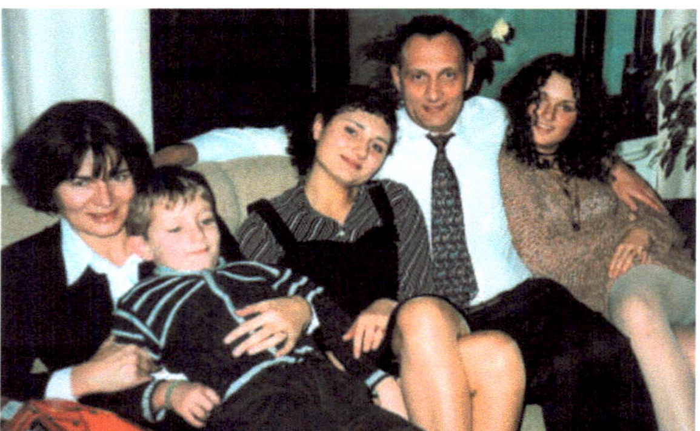

Joanna and Anna (son Adam came later), were not too happy about being uprooted from their new found affluence in the West. "But when I got back I was immediately made head of department and all the stupid obstacles were removed. Within a year or two, all the problems of contact with the West were almost completely solved. There are still big differences, but I feel a real European now."

Visitors to Gdansk please note: there is a new airport able to whisk Jassem anywhere in Europe in a few hours – and likewise travellers into Gdansk (and the September lung conference). While in the city, fellow oncologists could usefully visit Jassem's department, which after 14 years under his direction is now a major contributor to clinical trials: "Many patients are on protocols – we have around 30 clinical studies running here at present," he says.

A current study that Jassem highlights was designed by one of his junior assistants, Dr Rafal Dziadziuszko. "This addresses the impact of one of the cyclooxygenase-2 (COX-2) inhibitors administered in addition to pulmonary resection in non-small cell lung cancer," he says. "It was initiated here and is being run in about 20 institutions in central Europe. The EORTC Lung Cancer Group will also be joining the study."

As Jassem points out, cancer centres in central and eastern Europe have become "very efficient partners with good quality data," despite initial caution from organisations in the West. In fact, his first international cooperative moves were within central and eastern Europe – he was involved in the Cen-tral and Eastern European Oncology Group (CEEOG), which he now chairs. CEEOG was set up by another of Jassem's mentors, professor Sandor Eckhardt from the National Cancer Institute in Budapest, in the early 1980s. The group had regular meetings in Budapest – much easier to get to from Poland.

Jassem uses the word "efficient" a lot – as he says, cancer centres in the former Iron Curtain countries have not exactly been spoilt with hundreds of research proposals from industry and other bodies, and as a result members of the CEEOG have made the most of the protocols they have worked on. The work has paid off: "We are very satisfied. For example, our group has recently participated in a very large breast cancer protocol, and we contributed the largest number of patients."

Cancer centres in central and eastern Europe have become "very efficient partners with good quality data."

Apart from covering two oncology disciplines, Jassem also specialises in breast and lung cancer – this is no mean feat, even for a doctor

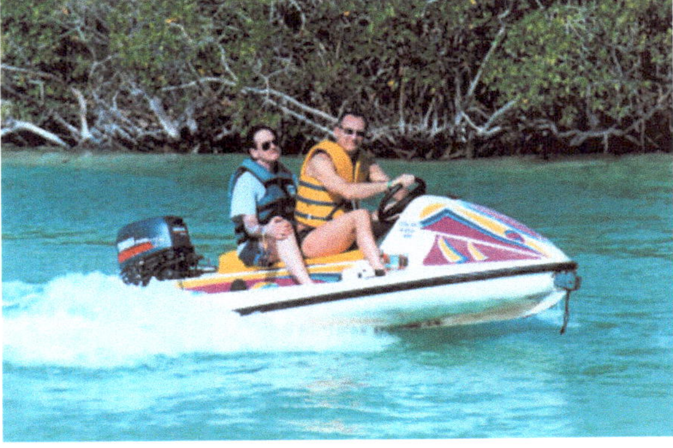

Speeding up the mouth of the river in Cancun, Mexico, with friend Professor Richard Gralla from the Columbia Medical Centre in New York. Jassem's holidays always involve plenty of action

of his energy. Work on lung cancer came first, but his interest in breast cancer arose both from it being the most common malignancy in Poland and the "fascinating changes in philosophy in treatment that has moved towards multidisciplinary therapies and breast preservation – this affected me a lot."

Wearing his international hat, Jassem weighs up the two worlds of breast and lung cancer and considers lung rather the poor relation in terms of large clinical studies. As he says, to find often small differences in outcomes there is a need for organisations such as the Breast Cancer Intergroup (BIG), the consortium that has around 30 cooperative groups capable of mounting studies with many thousands of patients. "That's an example of good international cooperation – but I'm not happy about the situation with lung cancer. We badly need such a structure for this disease, but organising and funding such a big enterprise is very difficult. We need similar global structures for other major malignancies such as head and neck, and colorectal cancer, as well."

Although highly cautious of the word "breakthrough," Jassem expects new learning about the molecular features of cancer cells to yield a "real chance for oncology" in the next ten years. And the challenge of finding out why some patients with the same tumour respond differently to treatment – and working up individualised therapies – is keeping his interest in oncology as fresh as ever. "I feel like Alice in Wonderland – on the other side of the mirror," he jokes. "But even with existing treatments we can probably do much more," he adds.

Jassem is also an academic teacher of some 30 years standing, and as a result, giving papers at large conferences is meat and drink to him. As a teacher, he tries to foster partnerships with his assistants and students, noting the rather paternalistic attitude of some senior counterparts in other countries.

He also promotes visits abroad for his assistants to leading cancer centres: "They come back with fantastic feedback, not only on new therapies but also with suggestions on how to organise the department better and improve the quality of treatment." His staff say he is quick to credit them for work they have carried out, and he has attracted a young team to the department – the average age is significantly less than in other Polish hospitals. A research meeting takes place each week, and Jassem argues that having many colleagues who are also active at international level is keeping Gdansk Medical University as one of the top cancer research centres in Poland – it's one of the few from the country to be active in the EU's Sixth Framework programme, for example.

Jassem's teaching doesn't end within the profession – for some time he's been one of Poland's leading medical faces in the mass media, giving interviews and making television programmes on health promotion topics, specifically those related to cancer prevention.

One TV series that Jassem helped to produce on health topics ran for two years in Poland. There still is, he says, a considerable barrier to break down about cancer. "You have to realise that here cancer is a taboo. Many people don't believe you can be cured – that it is always a nightmare and leads to death.”

Most recently Jassem's team has also organised a local concert highlighting cancer issues in Gdansk, which attracted several thousand people. Apart from performance artists, some of his cancer patients who were successfully treated stood up and gave short talks. "Cancer survivors are not that enthusiastic to talk about their disease, so this wasn't easy," he comments.

"You have to realise that here cancer is a taboo."

He is also an advocate of doctors involving patients much more with their treatment. "We have to convince other physicians that decisions should be taken with their patients, and that being treated within a new protocol is not a punishment but a great chance to be treated better than standard care. This is also a message we've tried to sell to the media – in women's magazines, for example – that people should be asking questions about new protocols that are available."

Polish doctors have also made surprisingly successful headway with their government on anti-smoking measures. "You won't see the Marlboro man on our streets now, nor at sporting events, and there are no cigarette vending machines," he says. That's because a few years ago all 460 Polish members of parliament were lobbied by doctors – Jassem personally visited 18 MPs – to convince them to pass anti-tobacco legislation.

"We said to them that after many years of communism this is not a healthy society. The people have bad habits: they drink and smoke too much, and have poor diets and so on – you as an MP have responsibility for the health problems."

Poland has now seen a rapid decrease in smoking rates, particularly among young men, and rates of lung cancer have levelled out after several decades of rapid increase. You won't be able to smoke at Gdansk airport, thanks to Jassem and his colleagues.

"After many years of communism this is not a healthy society."

To give messages on healthy lifestyles it is much better to practise what you preach – and Jassem does just that. This is a man who plays basketball religiously every Tuesday and Friday night – and woe betide anyone who interrupts this schedule. Indeed, his trips abroad are geared

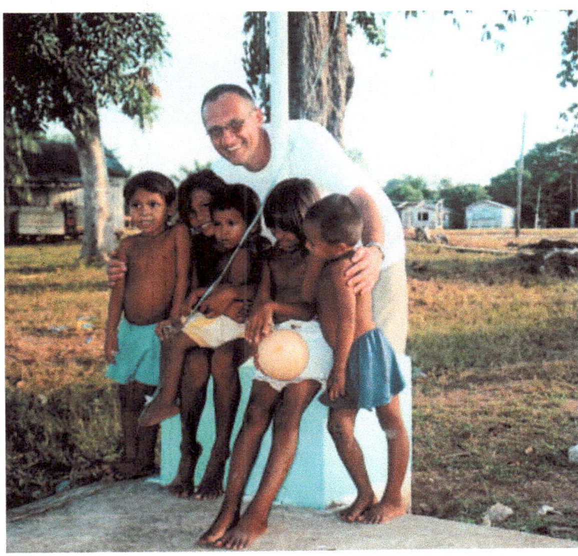

Having been confined to base in his early career, Jassem now makes the most of his travels abroad. This picture was taken in a village in the Amazon jungle that he visited when in Brazil for an oncology congress

around his amateur team matches in Gdansk.

At home (a house, incidentally, he helped to build himself), he has a fully equipped fitness room, and he and his family are all proficient skiers (Italy's Dolomites being the preferred destination for skiing holidays each year). The Jassem family certainly could have invented the term "activity holiday." Jassem is very unlikely to be spotted on a sun lounger – more likely on a canoe or windsurfer.

"Physical activity should be part of a daily schedule," says Jassem. "It gives me a feeling of wellbeing and makes me happy – my wife says that despite sometimes picking up small injuries I'm always very happy after basketball whether I win or lose." He's also a qualified mountain guide, and ran the student travel club in earlier days.

This work hard, play hard attitude – Jassem can spend up to 12 hours a day at the hospital, including weekends – is keeping him on top of a punishing schedule that also involves a large amount of travel. It's not unusual for Jassem to speak at a conference in Europe and make it back to Gdansk in time for a basketball match. If you send him an e-mail the chances are you'll get a reply within an hour or so, round the clock.

One of his daughters, Joanna, is following in her parents' footsteps and training in medicine, but she's heard enough conversations about lung cancer over dinner to put her off oncology – plastic surgery is her aim at present. The other daughter, Anna, is now a postgraduate student of politics at the European College in Bruges, Belgium; son Adam is 11 but has already travelled alone to England to boost his language skills.

Family members and assistants at the hospital describe Jassem, not surprisingly, as enormously energetic, committed and very hardworking in both professional and private life. He's no longer a party political animal – his work keeps him far too busy – but one senses similar organisational ability and leadership in the "politics" of cancer.

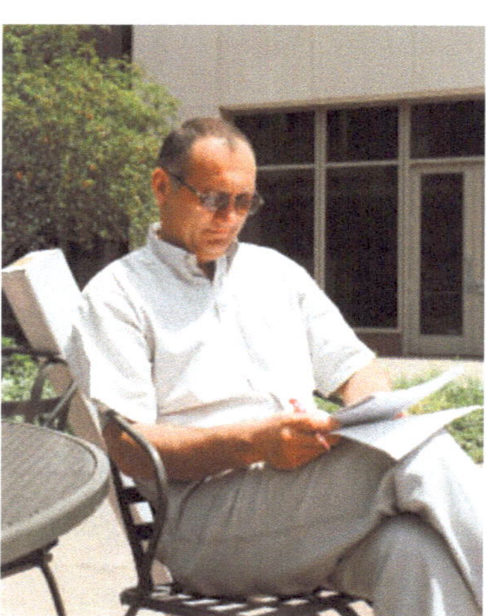

Preparing to deliver a paper at an ASCO meeting

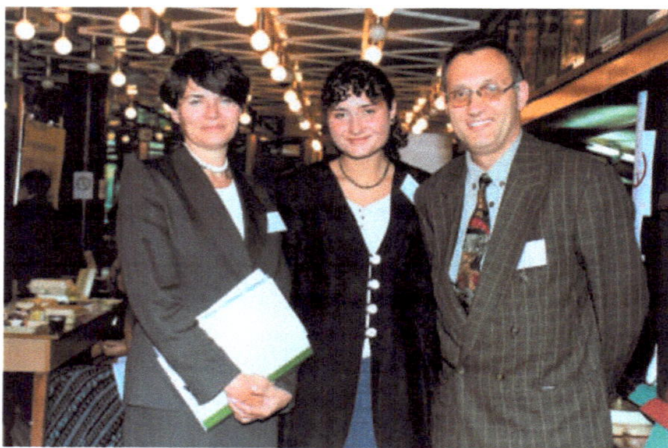

With his wife Ewa and older daughter Anna at an international lung cancer congress in Gdansk, October 2000. Anna, then a student of sociology, is about to make her first public presentation – on tobacco advertising policy in Poland

His dream for the near future is to build that dedicated cancer centre for Gdansk.

There's no switching off though at home – evening calls from terminally ill patients are said to "affect him deeply," no doubt only reinforcing the focus and single-mindedness he brings to his work.

His dream for the near future is to build that dedicated cancer centre for Gdansk. "I'm very happy with what I've achieved in my professional and family life, but we badly need a comprehensive cancer centre here – my team can't do any more with the facilities they've got."

This isn't necessarily a new building – although new equipment is of course needed – but a "structure where we can realise our professional plans: the potential of people here is very high." As he adds, Poland's survival rates for lung cancer are still poor in comparison with other European countries: "We need to prove we can translate our work into increased cure rates."

Investors take note – Jassem is likely to repay your commitment ten-fold.

Masterpieces

Interview with Umberto Veronesi

Maurice Schneider

Many oncologists have played a role in the astonishing developments in the field of cancer research and treatment in Europe over the past two decades. Few, however, can claim responsibility for shaping those developments, for having the vision to see what structures were needed to make best use of the rapid advances in knowledge, and having the drive to put them place. Such a one is Professor Veronesi. This celebrated Italian oncologist is the founding father of the European School of Oncology, the first institution to offer continuing medical education to Europe's cancer specialists, and is also responsible for the world-renowned European Oncology Institute in Milan. His determination to create the best conditions for progress in healthcare even led him to taking on the position of Minister for Health for a period. He remains, however, deeply involved in the cutting edge of cancer research, currently pushing forward investigations in the areas of breast and skin cancer. CancerFutures editor Maurice Schneider caught up with him in Milan, and asked him about his many areas of work.

Maurice Schneider: **The European School of Oncology has become a worldwide success in the 20 years since you founded it. What plans do you have for it now?**

Umberto Veronesi: At the time I founded the European School of Oncology, I felt that science was evolving at such a pace that doctors in Europe urgently needed a way to keep up to date with developments. The gap between new information becoming available and patients being able to benefit from that information was too long. We're talking about anything between five and seven years, and this was something our service found very disturbing.

So ESO began by spreading the word around about setting up as many courses as possible. Groups were organised by region, each with their own offices, and the progress has been tremendous – mainly due to the Director of ESO, Alberto Costa. He's an organisational genius!

In additional to running these courses, ESO is now looking to create some means of being affiliated to universities or institutes of research to do more in-depth and extended projects – a Masters degree in cancer of the breast, or of the prostate, for instance, or a Master in other fields, with a six months permanent course for people with a residency period in an important unit of certain hospitals. Of course, this is a totally new

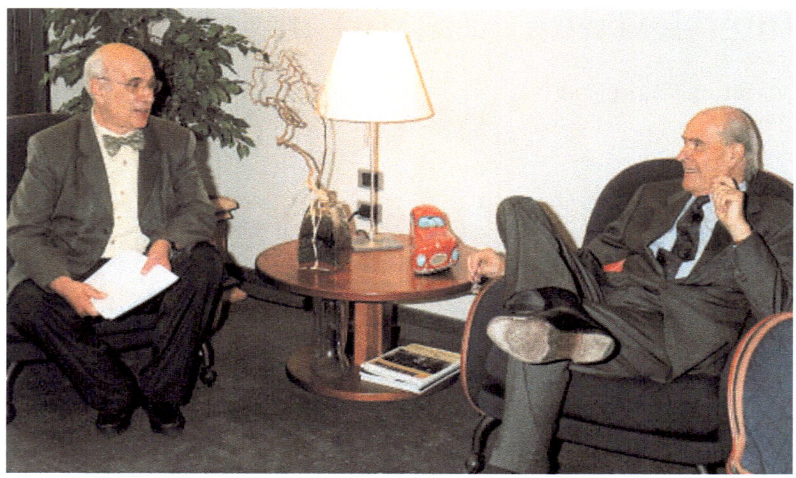

Prof. Umberto Veronesi (right) with the editor-in-chief of Cancer Futures, Prof. Maurice Schneider

approach for ESO. It demands a much more complicated organisational set-up – but I think this approach may constitute the second phase of the development of ESO.

The problem is to find a hospital that will accept these projects within their structures. I first have to approach the hospital and say, for instance: "I would like to use your urologic unit, to have our fellows work there for six months. We will discuss together a programme, and at the end you will provide them with a Masters degree". This is a big request, because the specialist titles we have in Europe, for instance in oncology or medical oncology, currently operate only at a higher level – there is no intermediate type of certification.

MS: I was very impressed by my visit to your European Oncology Institute in Milan. What is your policy now for the development of this Institute?

UV: Setting up the European Institute of Oncology was always going to be a challenge. Nobody believed that I would succeed in developing an institute that differed from the others in its fundamental principles: a different concept of patient care and an insistence on a high level of integration between laboratory research and clinical research. This institute is really European. We have members from fourteen countries working here, and having a large portion of the staff coming from outside Italy is a constitutional requirement. We speak English when we work, when we have our meetings. So it's a real European Institute. This was something totally new – there are no other examples in Europe. I think it provides a good way to integrate various colleagues, a cross-fertilisation of ideas between members coming from different European schools of oncology research.

MS: Where do your patients come from?

UV: The Institute treats many patients from many parts of Europe, although the majority are, of course,

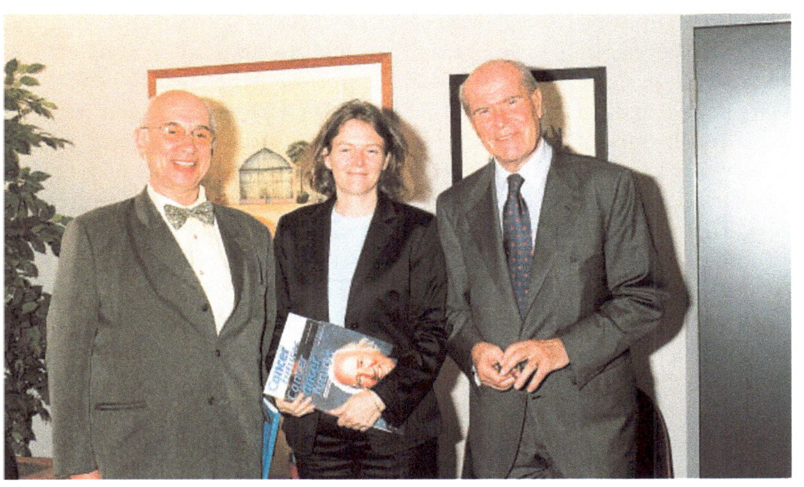

From left to right:
Prof. Maurice
Schneider,
Stéphanie
van Duin, director
of Springer-Verlag
France,
Prof. Umberto
Veronesi

Italians. The EOI developed so fast that it immediately established itself at the forefront of research, and this was perceived by the politicians and by the population, so we are swamped not only by patients, but also by fellows and researchers.

MS: Unusually for an oncology surgeon, you have also had the chance to formulate health policy when you served as Minister of Health. What was that like?

UV: That's a difficult question. I was probably too ambitious when I took over as Minister of Health. I had a very large number of projects I wanted to see implemented. If you have too many projects, you won't be able to see them all through in one year. Many of them end up just being discussed in Parliament, but never getting approval because they run out of time. The first law I worked on was probably the most effective – it was designed to protect non-smokers, by insisting that in offices, restaurants and anywhere, if you smoke you must do so in a separate area. This very simple law, very logical, very well received, didn't make it through Parliament. A large number of amendments were discussed, and finally it just failed to reach the statute book. I did, on the other hand, succeed in having a proposal accepted by the Parliament on liberalising the controlled use of opioids. Morphine, for instance, is not used very much in Italy, partly because doctors are concerned about the risk of addiction and also because they are afraid that somebody may use the prescription for other uses – not for medical use. However, we have to face the problem that a number of patients suffer very severe pain. Thanks to the law I introduced, doctors are now able to prescribe morphine without too much difficulty. This change in the law has been very beneficial, and was very well received by the population. Regarding progress in areas unrelated to cancer, of course there were plenty of projects. One was a greater freedom to use frozen embryos for terminal cell research, as in the UK. However, this measure met with very fierce opposition from the church. So fierce, in fact, that we were unable to proceed.

Another important law that was passed was to make continual medical education compulsory for all doctors. That was approved and is now in force. At the end of the year, all doctors in Italy now have to present 50 credit points, which they can earn by going to specific courses, or university seminars or congresses, or whatever. This is similar to the American system. These are the major issues arising out of my term as Minister of Health; there are plenty of other minor points but these are the most important.

MS: Did you enjoy your period in the Ministry of Health?

UV: I did and I didn't! I enjoyed it because you have the pleasure of creating projects, developing new ideas and working in a good environment. Ministries in Italy, at least the Ministry of Health, are full of very motivated officers, very intelligent, very active. People tend to get the impression that they don't work – it's not true – they work! I am a surgeon so I was accustomed to going to the office of the Minister of Health at 7 o'clock in the morning. At the beginning it was a shock for the employees, then by the end of the first week, at 7 o'clock everybody was there, and they stayed there till the end of the day – 7 o'clock at night. It was pleasant to participate in the development of important political decisions. The problem is that it is very difficult for a non-politician to interact with these politicians, because they inhabit differ-

ent worlds: it's a different language, politicians have different objectives, their main problem is to be re-elected next time. I discovered immediately that the main problem was not the well-being of the country – this is important, but it is the second objective, not the first. First of all – be re-elected; look for a good consensus among the population, so as to get into government, to remain in the government, to win the elections ... This is the obsession of politicians everywhere in the world. Inside this framework, of course, you may have other important objectives, but for me it was difficult to understand why certain proposals were accepted and others were rejected, without a logical reasoning – at least not one that made sense within my philosophy.

MS: I would now like to turn to your research into the use of the sentinel node biopsy procedure in breast cancer. Tell me something about the results so far

UV: This research started many years ago, because we were not certain whether the axillary spread of breast cancer would provide good anatomical conditions for diagnosis by the sentinel node biopsy. The procedure was introduced for diagnosing melanoma, and in this context it proved to be effective. But for the breast, we wanted to establish whether distribution of the cancer cells in the axilla would be appropriate for using the sentinel biopsy procedure.

So we conducted a long study on 1500 patients, mapping all the nodes one by one, and in the end we concluded that the spreading axilla of the cancer cells coming from the breast is a regular spread. This research was carried out between 1985 and 1995. In 1995, we decided to start using the sentinel node biopsy procedure at this Institute. We started with a validation study, which showed that we were able to make a correct diagnosis of the axilla involvement, by taking the sentinel node alone, in 96.8% of the cases. So the accuracy was 96.8% and the rate of false-negatives was 3.2%. A 3% false-negative rate is acceptable – it's not very high – but we have to be aware of the possibility and we have to inform women of this very tiny risk.

After this validation study, we randomised 516 patients into two groups, exactly divided. One group received the sentinel biopsy and axillary dissection, the other group received the sentinel biopsy and, if it proved negative, no axillary dissection. We concluded this study in 1999, and we have now completed nearly 4 years' follow-up. For the moment, the two groups are doing more or less the same, but the group with the sentinel node biopsy only is doing slightly better. We lost two patients in this group, compared to five patients in the axillary dissection group.

This is very encouraging, we don't know what will happen over the next 3 or 4 years, but it looks like the projection is favourable. That initial result gave us confidence. We are now offering sentinel biopsies to all women as a routine practice, and we have carried out more than 3000 such procedures. We are very happy, the patients are very happy, the costs have been much reduced, our hospitalisation period is very short – one day, maybe two for an important cancer – and in my opinion, this will be the future of breast cancer surgery.

MS: Finally, I'd like to ask you where we are now concerning research into melanoma?

UV: I think melanoma is a disease that needs two different approaches.

The first one is to find a means of early detection. A number of projects have been developed for naevi mapping, very sophisticated, with a great number of variables in the computer. Once these are in place, then you'll be able to screen and to see whether naevi are normal or suspicious for development. This bio-informatic progress is very important, because if we can evaluate everyone with a periodic mapping, with these very beautiful, fantastic machines, we could really achieve a very early detection of melanoma. And very early melanoma is cured in 99% of the cases; it's not a very serious disease when spotted very early.

The other approach is the immunological approach. Melanoma is, of course, probably one of the only tumours with specific antigens. We have to make use of this information and put in motion large studies with vaccines or with the specific antibodies. This is the future of the projects in progress. For the moment the results are not very strong, but a number of responses are there. There are a number of cases where the melanomas have just disappeared. They are not very many, but something is there. We must insist on finding the key, the final key to the solution.

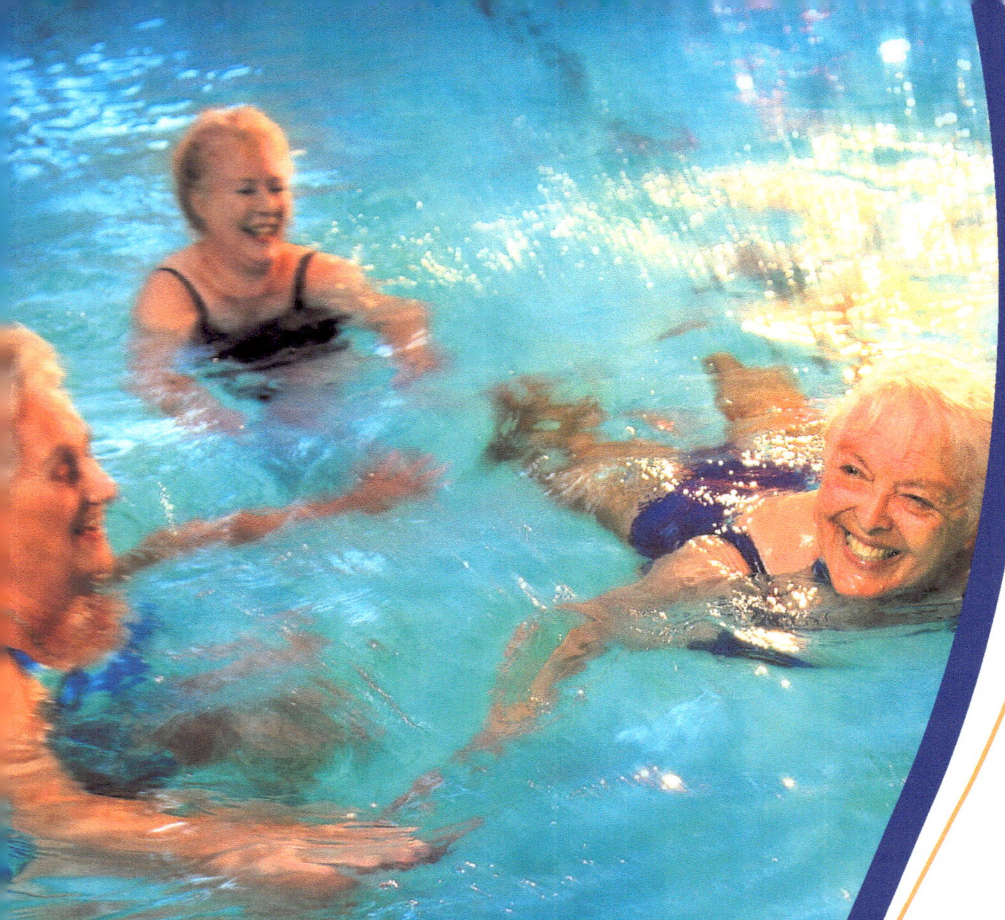

'Faslodex' provides
your postmenopausal
patients with an effective
once-monthly treatment
so they can focus on their
lives, not their illness.

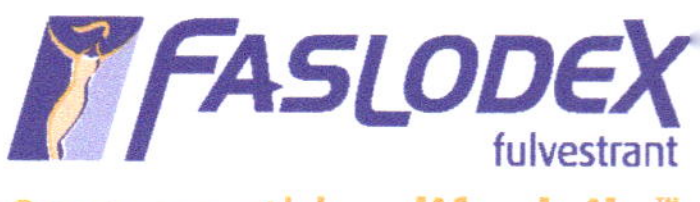

The first and only estrogen receptor antagonist
with no agonist effects for the treatment of
advanced breast cancer

'Faslodex' and 'Faslodex' logo are trademarks
of the AstraZeneca group of companies

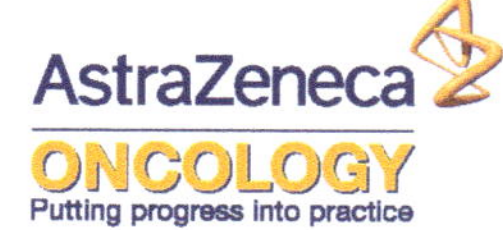

8288/October 2004

Maurice Tubiana:
The Fighting Spirit Behind Cancerology

MAURICE SCHNEIDER and RAPHAËL BRENNER

A pioneer in cancer therapy, French oncologist Professor Maurice Tubiana, member of the French Academy of Sciences and Academy of Medicine, and former head of the Gustave Roussy Institute in Villejuif, France, personally took part in the revolution in biological knowledge that led to modern biomedicine. In conversation with Maurice Schneider and Raphaël Brenner of CancerFutures, Professor Tubiana looks back on a life full of hope and achievement.

CancerFutures: **You dealt with cancer and with death throughout your life. Do you fear old age and the prospect of death?**

Maurice Tubiana: I have just spent the last two years writing a book about old age [Le bien vieillir, De Fallois]. As a man over 80, living in a society that is intolerant towards the old and can even brutally reject them, I cannot ignore the fact that it is difficult to be old. The first time I became aware of this was when I was still head of the Gustave Roussy Institute. I was driving to work one day when, at a red light, a man in the car next to me opened his window and said: "Hey, grandpa, why are you dawdling? You're annoying those who are going to work. Move over to the side and give way." The truth is that old people symbolise what's going to happen to all of us – we are all going to get old and die, and young people don't want to be reminded of this. They want to get rid of the old or at least shove them away from view.

As far as I am concerned, old age is fine. I write, I read Camus and philosophers like Montaigne and Pascal, and through them I understand that nothing is worse than idleness. Montaigne wrote that he would like to die "while planting his cabbages." In other words, having a daily activity and interests enables us to ward off death. This is what I try to do. My curiosity in the world around me has not diminished.

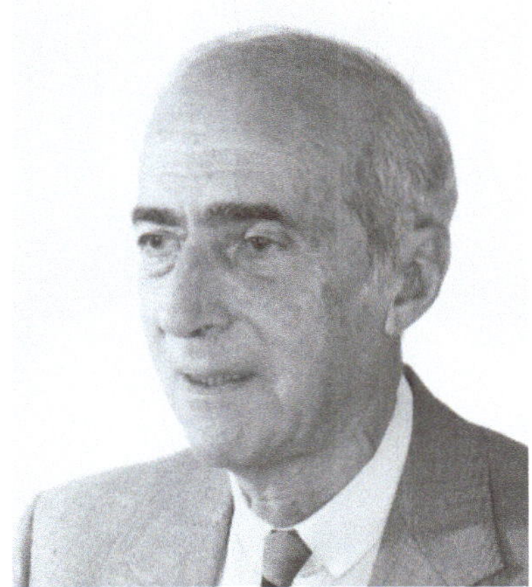

CF: How did you become a physician and researcher?

MT: I grew up in Algeria, in a strongly observant Jewish family, where I learnt to respect intellectual activities, and this had a major influence on my choice of career. My family gave me a taste for study, and this in turn gave me a taste for research. The other factor that influenced me was the deep significance of the Day of Atonement. This is one time in the year when we look back and ask: "What have I done with my life?" I remember my father telling me when I was just six or seven: "You have all day to think about what you've done in the last year. Think about it seriously and think about it again every year." This had a profound effect on me. Every year, I ask myself: what did I do with my life in the last year and what do I intend to do with my life? This reminds me of Tolstoy, who wrote in Confessions: "I'm rich, very rich. So what? I am one of the greatest Russian writers. So what? What have I done with my life?"

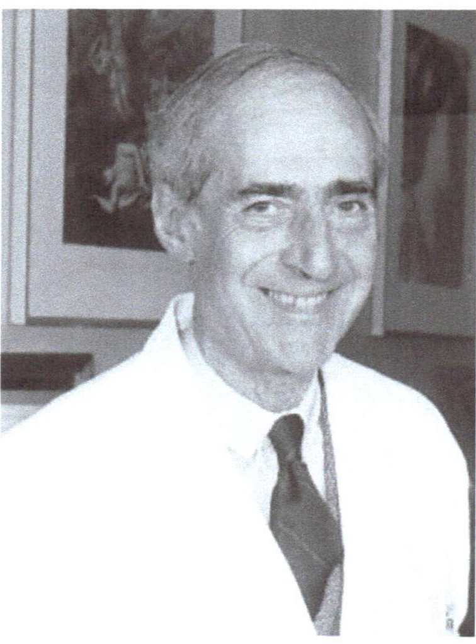

CF: What have you done with your life?

MT: As a Jew I lived under a false identity during the war in occupied France. Then, in 1943, I joined the Free French Forces in Algeria and participated in the Italian campaign. The war deeply influenced my life because it gave me a taste for action and, paradoxically, it was the happiest period of my life. I needed to fight an enemy, and this is why I found cancerology so attractive. I also have a taste for facts. In Algeria, I grew up in an environment immersed in superstition and irrationality. Faced with so much irrationality, I became fascinated by science and by reason, which seemed to me to be good counterweights and to hold the key to the future and to progress. I remember reading Jules Verne's Mystery Island when I was a child, and this is still the book that most influenced me. I craved rationality and found it in modern medicine. So after the war, I started to work in the laboratory of Frédéric Joliot-Curie, and this is how I came to specialise in radioactive isotopes. In 1947, I went to the US to do research at Berkeley. It was wonderfully stimulating. Just as in Mystery Island, the combination of scientific and social aspects have always been essential in my life.

CF: You have contributed to many advances in cancerology: radiotherapy of lymphomas and thyroid carcinomas, the application of nuclear medicine, and radiobiology. What gave you the most satisfaction?

MT: It's true that I dabbled in many fields and derived a lot of pleasure and satisfaction out of everything I did. But I would say that what gave me the greatest pleasure is the human dimension – the contact I had with my students and fellow workers. I remember that we had two staff meetings every week and this was, for me, the best time of the week. There is no doubt that I find great satisfaction in being a teacher, having young people around me, talking with them and helping them in their professional choices.

CF: Which discoveries do you consider were milestones in cancer therapy during your career?

MT: Two events changed my life. First, the introduction of cobalt as a means of high-energy radiation in 1953. Results of treatment were very poor until then. Then, suddenly, we had a highly effective radioisotope at our disposal and everything changed. It was a very exciting time. We found a new therapeutic application almost every month. The other very exciting event took place in 1963 when the British Medical Journal published an article demonstrating that it was possible to cure Hodgkin's disease. This was a revelation. I remember Jean Bernard being very sceptical about the article. He called me, saying: "What's all this talk about a cure for Hodgkin's disease? It must be a mistake on the part of cytologists." "Perhaps," I answered, "but perhaps it's true." Then we started to study the issue and to establish new treatments, and from an 8–10% success rate at the beginning, we went on to achieve success rates of 80–85% within 15 years for patients suffering from Hodgkin's disease. What was

also innovative was that it was the first time in cancer therapy that we used a multi-disciplinary approach for the treatment and, even more importantly, we systematically used quantitative clinical trials involving comparisons and randomisations.

CF: How do you assess your role as health adviser to the French government and as a cancer policy maker in Europe?

MT: This was a very challenging role, and I believe we demonstrated that a wide-scale campaign against cancer is possible. In 1985, President

"I needed an enemy to fight and this is why I found cancerology so attractive."

Mitterand asked me, together with other specialists, to propose a health programme at a European level. He felt that Europe was considered solely as an economic union and he wanted to show that Europe could also bring many improvements to peoples' lives. So we decided to establish the "European Campaign Against Cancer." This is how Italian cancerologist Umberto Veronesi and I came to work together on this project, of which I was the director. The British and the Germans were extremely sceptical about such a project. So we focused the programme on prevention and early screening.

CF: Why the focus on prevention?

MT: From my time at the CIRC [International Centre for Cancer Research] in Lyon, I knew that more than 50% of deaths due to cancer could be avoided with appropriate prevention. So we launched a major campaign against smoking. We anticipated a 15% reduction in the death rate from tobacco-induced cancers in Europe. The rate fell by 9% between 1986 and 2000, which is still good. In any case, I am pleased to see that everyone acknowledges

"We need a strong European Authority to implement laws for safeguarding health."

today that fighting cancer means fighting smoking. But I remain cautious about laws and regulations, because the important thing is not the actual law but its implementation. We still have a long way to go. The wealth and power of the tobacco industry is enormous; it has the best lawyers and the best psychologists. This is the reason why Europe must take effective action against the tobacco industry.

CF: Do you think that Europe is relevant in the field of health?

MT: Definitely, I think Europe has an essential role to play in this field. The three main causes of cancer and other severe diseases in Europe are: smoking, alcohol and overeating, and no campaign against any of these factors is possible without a concerted European strategy. Take the problem of smoking. If you ban advertising of cigarettes or increase the price of cigarettes in only one European country, it's useless, because people can purchase cigarettes, buy newspapers or watch TV from other countries. So it's essential to act on a European scale and we need a strong European Authority to implement laws for safeguarding health. In actual fact, in order to implement health policies, we need to have a European FDA and CDC [Food and Drug Administration and Centers for Disease Control and Prevention, in the US]. Until such a time, there can be no such thing as European health.

Michael Baum: Shooting Sacred Cows

Helen Saul

Professor Michael Baum is Professor Emeritus of Surgery and visiting Professor of Medical Humanities at University College, London. He was one of the instigators of both the IBIS (International Breast Cancer Intervention Study) and ATAC (Arimidex, Tamoxifen, Alone or in Combination) trials, and has won numerous awards for his work, including two for a life-time achievement in breast cancer research – the Miami Breast Cancer conference award, 2001, and the William McGuire award, San Antonio, 2002 – and, also in 2002, the American Society of Clinical Oncology's Best of Oncology Award for the best contribution over the previous 12 months.

CancerFutures: How did IBIS come to be set up?

Michael Baum: I was the principal investigator of the Cancer Research Campaign tamoxifen adjuvant trials, and our group was the first to show the benefits of tamoxifen. As a spin-off, the statistician Jack Cuzick, with whom I have worked for decades, and I noted a significant reduction in contralateral cancer among tamoxifen-treated patients. This, along with laboratory data from Craig Jordan's laboratory, made us think that tamoxifen had potential for the prevention of breast cancer. But using it in prevention as opposed to in treatment poses an enormous ethical dilemma. If in any one year, two women in 1,000 get breast cancer, and you have a good treatment which halves that risk, it means that for every one breast cancer you prevent in any one year, 999 women are exposed to the side-effects of the drug.

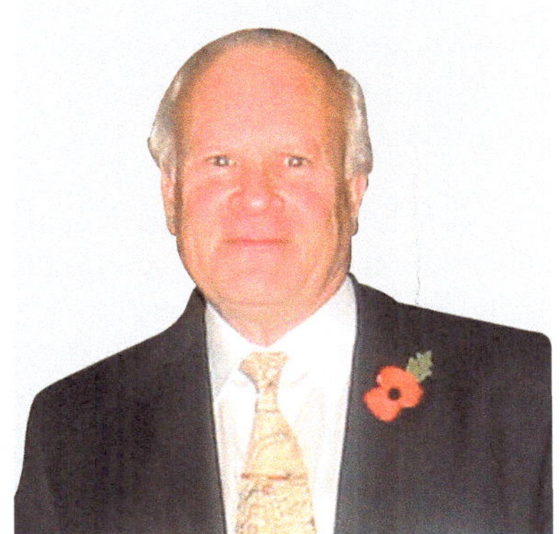

At the same time, we thought tamoxifen had favourable side effects and could prevent osteoporosis and protect against ischaemic heart disease. On balance, the benefits might outweigh the harms and it justified a large-scale multicentre trial. IBIS was the first, but four other trials were established. By 2002, we had proof of principle, but in my judgement and in Jack Cuzick's, no good evidence of clinical efficacy. The overview of the five prevention trials showed undoubtedly that tamoxifen can reduce the incidence of oestrogen-receptor-positive breast cancers. But the IBIS study, to my mind, found unacceptable adverse events, particularly thromboembolism, and the net effect on all-cause mortality was zero.

It's now down to qualitative interpretation of the data. The Americans feel there are enough data to advocate tamoxifen prevention for high-risk women, but on this side of the Atlantic, and certainly this is my feeling, although there is proof of principle, I cannot advocate it as standard therapy.

CF: The discrepancy is interesting, particularly as the women in the European trials were probably at higher risk of breast cancer than those in the US trials

MB: There is a paradox here: the higher the risk of the group, the more likely they are to have a genetic predisposition and the more likely to be at risk of oestrogen-receptor-negative tumours. They are therefore less likely to benefit from tamoxifen. I don't think that's the end of chemoprevention; in the ATAC trial, we recently reported that anastrozole was significantly better in delaying or preventing breast cancer than tamoxifen, so aromatase inhibitors may be a better bet for the prevention of breast cancer than tamoxifen.

IBIS II has been launched with anastrozole versus a placebo control, and tamoxifen has been dropped (I have stepped down from the IBIS committee now). A lot of work is going on into selecting new agents, but

I think we have promising agents, it's just that we are using them on unselected populations. We need to be much more selective, and there is increasing sophistication in predicting groups at high risk for developing hormone-receptor-positive breast cancers. But it may be another 10 years before we have anything sufficiently important to advocate policy changes.

The subject is by no means dead. The Americans are comparing raloxifene with tamoxifen, but my personal prejudice is that we are more likely to see progress through better treatment than primary or secondary prevention.

CF: Did the IBIS results come as a great disappointment?

MB: Not really. I've seen it through from hypothesis generation to proof of principle and, as a clinical scientist, I'm thrilled. But a clinical scientist has also got to make judgements about benefits versus harms.

CF: How is it that populations on opposite sides of the Atlantic can look at the same data and come to different conclusions?

MB: There are enormous cultural differences, among both patients and clinicians. American culture is driven by a fear of litigation, which makes for a lot of defensive medicine. The rights of the individual are centre stage; individuals feel empowered to access the Internet and demand what they think is appropriate. In Europe, patients tend to be more passive and clinicians tend to be less defensive.

CF: On screening – you were involved in setting up a screening programme in London, but you're now a vocal critic. Did you change your mind over time, or were you always sceptical?

MB: A good scientist has to start from a position of scepticism, but in 1987 I was prepared to accept that there were sufficient data showing that screening could reduce breast cancer mortality. I was given the task of setting up one of the first screening programmes in the country when I was Professor of Surgery at King's College London. I took enormous pride in setting this up, together with the Head of Radiology. We built a beautiful centre to serve South East London and a training unit for the South East of England. I was appointed to the National Screening Committee.

But I became more and more disillusioned with screening as I learnt first hand about its toxic side effects. Unlike radiologists or epidemiologists, a surgeon picks up the pieces. I saw all the terror of the false-positives, the unnecessary surgery, the endless discussions on borderline pathology: was it atypical ductal hyperplasia, was it ductal carcinoma in situ (DCIS)? The dismay for women turning up, thinking they were well, and being told they had DCIS. "You are lucky because it is early, but by the way you have to have a mastectomy because it is multifocal." I began to question whether the benefits outweighed the costs. Then I began to look at screening not in terms of relative risk reductions, but in terms of absolute benefits: how many women do you need to screen to stop

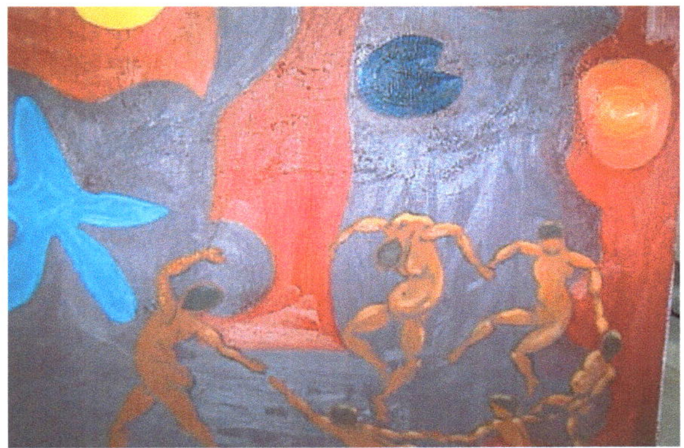

Michael Baum, Breaking the ring

one woman dying of breast cancer. I am not the only one to look at data in that way. The most reasonable estimate – the one that is accepted by the US task force on cancer prevention – is that 1,500 women have to be screened for 10 years to stop one woman dying of breast cancer. No one disputes that number. That woman's life is of infinite value. If we were talking about fluoridisation of the tap water, or wearing seat belts, fine, but we are not. We are talking about procedures with consequences. To my mind, the worst problem is the overdiagnosis of DCIS, a disease that we almost never saw, which now represents 20% of all incident cases. Anything between 30 to 40% of these women end up with a mastectomy.

CF: And you only have to have one suicide in the group, for example, to wipe out the benefit of screening?

MB: Exactly. I don't want to overstate the case, but as you've said it, yes. We are talking about cause-specific mortality. Compare that with chemoprevention. We can prevent 30 to 40% of breast cancers, but the side effects of tamoxifen make me question whether it is a wise choice. With screening, no one in the screening community is prepared to come out and say, "There may be adverse effects and it is not implausible that some of these adverse events could lead to at least one death in 15,000 women-years of screening." I find it absolutely arrogant that the screening community cannot accept that there is a downside to what they do. To my mind, the worst thing is that women are summoned for screening. This is almost fascistic. The screening community says their

"It shows enormous disrespect for women not to explain the downside as well as the upside of screening."

"invitations" include the information necessary. That's simply not true. The invitations are upbeat and say there is a 25% reduction in your risk of dying from breast cancer if you come for screening. Women are made to feel foolish if they don't accept screening. It shows enormous disrespect for women not to explain the downside as well as the upside. It's double standards. When we're inviting patients to have surgery, radiotherapy or chemotherapy, we do so with informed consent. We explain the benefits and the harms, and we try to use decision-making tools, which give benefits in absolute not relative terms. I do not see that ethical standard in screening.

CF: Yours is an unpopular point of view. Do you have any support?

MB: I have enormous support, but a lot of people are frightened to

raise their head above the parapet. It has not been pleasant to take a stand on this; I have been subjected to all kinds of abuse and vilification from the screening industry. I was once accused on television, by an epidemiologist, for being responsible for the death of one in every 1,000 women.

I recently published a paper on the subject in the British Medical Journal with Mrs Hazel Thornton, who is a lay advocate. Most of the online responses were hugely supportive. I suspect there's a silent majority out there who support this position, but individuals like me are up against an industry with a £50 million (572 million) turnover a year, plus the government of the day. The announcement that screening was to be introduced was made by Margaret Thatcher two weeks before the 1987 general election. It was used as a tool for political gain, and it would be political suicide for any government to decide to close down a screening programme.

Whenever you challenge dogma it is unpleasant, but if you don't, you don't advance the subject. There is proof of principle for screening, but the downside totally outweighs the benefits. And there's the issue of opportunity costs: £50 million a year spent on rapid access to specialist clinics and rapid access to radiotherapy would improve breast cancer mortality more than screening.

Screening is a last residual echo of the "catch it early and take it all away" dogma. The disease is much more complex than that, early cancer is latent cancer, and once latent cancer is triggered to become invasive cancer, the pattern of outcome is predetermined. We need fresh insights about the nature of the disease, and at the moment, many scientists at the cutting edge are evolving the conceptual model.

CF: Do you see your views on screening holding sway?

MB: No. At the moment the screening zealots have the loudest voice. They call consensus meetings to which they invite only believers, and they come up with consensus statements which state that the case for screening is proven, now let's move on. That expression, "Let's move on," intensely irritates me; they want to shut the door on further argument. The position should be "Let's think again," and probably the position I would like to get to is that the age group for screening changes. There would probably be more bangs for the buck, more sensitivity and specificity, if the age group was 55 to 69, rather than the 50 to 64 years. And surely it's not too much to ask that women give informed consent and are made aware of the downside when they are invited for screening. I would hope that consumer advocacy groups support me on that.

Looking ahead, screening has a great future behind it! People are now talking about MRI and other techniques, which may increase the sensitivity but decrease the specificity. MRIs show up a lot more latent lesions which it's probably best not to know about. I see no useful advances to be made in this direction; things can only get worse with the new imaging techniques.

CF: Moving on to treatment and your role in the ATAC trial, do the results mean tamoxifen has had its day?

MB: Not at all. To my mind, the greatest impact on breast cancer mortality has been adjuvant systemic therapy – and I say that as a surgeon. The first overview – the Early Breast Cancer Trials Collaborative Group overview in 1985 – was the seminal event. Certainly, in this country, mortality has decreased by about 30% since 1985, in spite of an increasing incidence. Most of that

"Screening has a great future behind it."

is attributable to better treatment, chemotherapy and hormonal therapy.

Combining treatments where appropriate is better than any one alone. And the most important thing is that oestrogen and progesterone receptors have emerged as powerful predictive tests in selecting patients. What we need now are new agents and better predictive factors.

I don't think for a moment that tamoxifen has had its day. We now have choice; just as there is a choice of chemotherapy regimens, we now have a choice of endocrine therapy regimens. As data emerges from the ATAC trial over the next few years and we look more closely at the biological profiles, I'm confident that we'll find two subgroups of hormone responsive breast cancers. One will do better with tamoxifen and the other with anastrozole. We can also look at the toxicity and tolerability profiles of patients, and choose the more appropriate treatment. So if the patient has osteoporosis or is at high risk of osteoporosis, tamoxifen may be favoured over anastrozole. By contrast, patients at high risk of thromboembolic disease and patients at risk of endometrial cancer would be better off with anastrozole than tamoxifen.

So for me, the excitement of the ATAC result is not that we have something to replace tamoxifen, it's that we have a choice. There may indeed be horses for courses.

The next formal analysis will be triggered statistically. The first formal analysis was triggered by the number of first events and the next update will be triggered statistically when we cross the threshold for distant disease-free survival and/or death. That analysis should set the seal on the subject.

There are on-going trials in which women have one agent and then switch, and we await the outcome with great interest. My concern is that ATAC has already shown that the curves separate in favour of anastrozole within three years. Patients on tamoxifen who then switch to anastrozole not only have to do better, but they have a lot of catching up to do.

CF: What advances have you seen in surgery over your career?

MB: I'm still a practising surgeon, but I find surgery the least interesting bit of breast cancer. In the early 1970s, though, when the young Turks around the world, led by Bernie Fisher in Pittsburgh, were challenging the dogma of radical mastectomy, it was very, very exciting. There was blood all over the floor. The prevailing anatomi-

cal dogma – that the disease starts in the breast, spreads centrifugally along the lymphatics and is arrested in the lymph nodes that act as filters protecting the body – had to be overturned. The assumption was false and led to radical treatment. Once the dogma was overturned, progress accelerated in all directions. The one thing we have got to learn from the past is that once everybody agrees that it is so, someone has got to have the courage to say, "Maybe not."

Everybody now accepts that breast-conserving surgery is a safe option, and even women who have to have a mastectomy have reconstruction. There's a lot of interest in sentinel node biopsy, which is a minor advance, but I'm more interested in the interface between surgery and radiotherapy. I've been involved in setting a trial of intraoperative radiotherapy, in which all the radiotherapy required is given at the time of surgery. The technology exists, phase I and phase II trials have been completed, and there are a number of phase III trials on-going. If they work out, it is a real advance and would mean women in the developing world can be offered breast conserving surgery. At the moment, if you live more than 100 miles away from a radiotherapy centre anywhere in the world, including USA or Australia, your chances of receiving breast conserving therapy are remote. So for parts of the Western world where distance is a factor and parts of the developing world where availability and cost is a factor, we will be able to offer more breast conserving surgery. It's an exciting marker for the future.

You remove the tumour, and insert a probe that can generate radiation into the cavity. You wrap the cavity wall around the probe, switch it on for half an hour, and irradiate with maximum dose 1–2 cm beyond the cavity wall. Surgeons are doing this; the specialisms of surgery and radiotherapy are merging. We will have to reconsider the training of breast surgeons. I think we need breast clinicians with surgical, medical and radiotherapy skills.

For the future, this technique may be combined with minimally invasive surgery. We have done a few cases where the tumour is cut away through a relatively small puncture wound, and the radiotherapy source inserted. It's entirely plausible that minimally invasive surgery plus radiotherapy could be given in a single session as an outpatient.

MB: I am a passionate scientist and will defend science to the death, but I am concerned that if you become totally obsessed with science, some of the humane aspects of medicine are lost. Along with many others, I pioneered programmes of medical humanities in medical schools, and I still teach a module on the history of art and the history of medicine. I aim to teach students to stand back and look at the generalities, to try to understand human suffering and what empathy means. You can't learn empathy down a microscope.

The subjects of art and medicine run in parallel throughout history, and in fact St Luke is the patron saint of both medicine and art. In Renais-

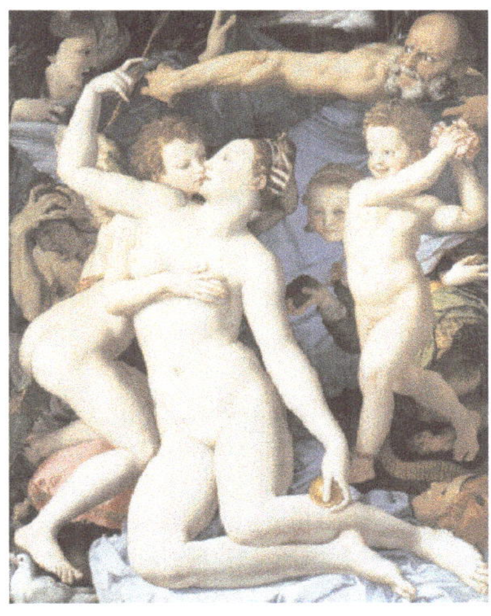

Agnolo Bronzino, An Allegory with Venus and Cupid

sance times, apothecaries and artists shared rooms, and in the 1800s John Hunter was professor of Anatomy at the Royal Academy of Art. There is a long tradition, and I'm keen on maintaining it.

You can learn a lot from interpreting paintings, and I always take my group round the National Gallery to look at wonderful old masterpieces and diagnose them. It's called iconology. All great paintings

"You can't learn empathy down a microscope."

have hidden messages, like signs and symptoms. Studying art teaches you about observation and deduction, and gives you a window on the soul. Art illustrates human suffering. Empathy means getting inside someone's head and looking out and you can only do that through fine literature, poetry, and fine art.

A wonderful painting by Agnolo Bronzino, An Allegory with Venus and Cupid, is an allegory of sacred and profane love. It had been assumed that this was full of iconography of venereal disease. But the year before last, my group of students not only identified all the stigma identified with syphilis, much of which had already been reported, but they made an original discovery. A cherub holding flowers is standing on a thorn which has penetrated his foot, and he is smiling beatifically. He has no sensation in his feet, which is a sign of tertiary syphilis. They spotted it. So, they learnt observation, deduction, diagnosis and they probably know more about tertiary syphilis than most of their teachers, because it encouraged them to go back to the textbooks and read about the subject.

Usually iconography means diagnosing the messages. Another powerful painting is The Ambassadors, by Hans Holbein. It's full of powerful, detailed iconography about the Reformation and the Counter-Reformation, the world turned upside down in the time of Henry VIII. Taking them through it teaches them to open their eyes, look for clues and translate them.

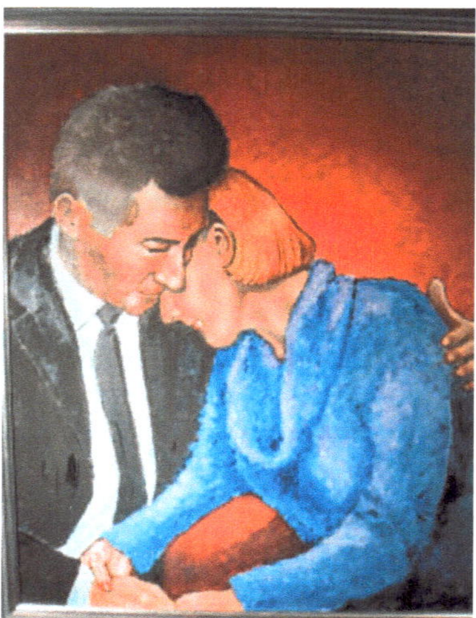

**Michael Baum,
The Consultation**

CF: You also paint?

MB: I have always dabbled and sketched, and I used to be the cartoonist for a student magazine. But I have spent a couple of years learning the craft with an artist, and I showed three works at the Mall Galleries in July 2003. My painting is not fashionable. One painting, for example, is called The Consultation, and it is of a woman who has just had a bad diagnosis, with her husband. She is a patient of mine, and she and her husband allowed me to take a photo re-enacting the diagnosis; I painted from the photo. A companion piece, Diptych: The Consultation, is a rather grim self-portrait. I'm back-lit, looking aloof and dispassionate. It's meant to portray the problem of true empathy, and convey the way the doctor is perceived by the patient.

Painting for me is cathartic, it is relaxation, using a different side of the brain, and it is therapeutic. I paint from life, portraits and nudes. Doctors compartmentalise the way they look at women, as a clinical object, separate from the way a red-blooded man sees a woman. In addition, through the eyes of an artist, I see women in another, different way. Painting a beautiful nude reminds you of what you do in the operating theatre, and it has always inspired me to look for nonsurgical techniques and ways of reducing surgical morbidity.

**CF: How do you see the future
of breast cancer?**

MB: I'd like to see the incidence go down not as a result of chemoprevention, but as a result of public health education and lifestyle choices. I'd like to see young women starting their families early, and keeping their weight down. I'd like to see less alcohol abuse amongst young women: these lifestyle choices could reverse the increasing incidence of the disease.

I'd like to see the morbidity of local treatment become less, and I would like to see more choice in therapy, so that treatments are tailored to the biological character of the cancer. That is not necessarily going to be through molecular biology, which has ignored important epigenetic aspects of cancer, such as the microvasculature, the nature of the physics by which cells orientate themselves and the physics by which the fractal geometry of the blood supply of the tumour is distorted. The answer isn't entirely genetic; that's another dogma we need to challenge. But I am optimistic that this type of progress is achievable over a 20-year period.

Hans-Jörg Senn: Championing Consensus

ANNA WAGSTAFF

Throughout his long career, Professor Hans-Jörg Senn of the St Gallen Tumour Detection and Prevention Centre has shown an impressive ability to keep one step ahead of the field. In 1972 he was among a small group who initiated one of the first trials of adjuvant treatment of breast cancer, despite heavy opposition from the wider medical oncology community, who thought it was crazy to give chemotherapy to healthy women. In the mid-1980s he was one of the first to recognise that the heady pace of progress in finding medical solutions to cancer was slowing down, and that it was up to oncologists to find ways to help their patients live with their disease. And today, Professor Senn's

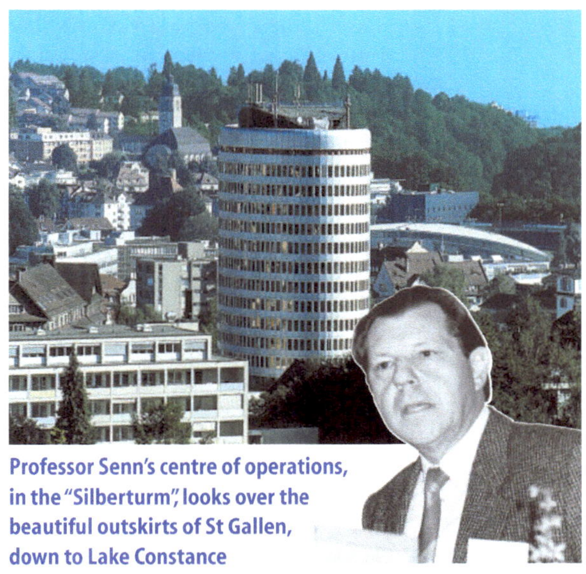

Professor Senn's centre of operations, in the "Silberturm", looks over the beautiful outskirts of St Gallen, down to Lake Constance

St Gallen centre is flagging up primary and secondary prevention as the next logical priority in the major cancers. It is a record that any budding young medical oncologist might wish to emulate. And yet, arguably, the unique talent of Professor Senn lies not so much in his pioneering ideas, but in his ability to bring the medical oncology community along with him. For it was from a small meeting in St Gallen of those "crazy" trialists that the International St Gallen Guidelines – now the reference point for adjuvant breast cancer therapy over much of the Western world – were later to emerge. How did he do it? Anna Wagstaff from CancerFutures took the train to St Gallen to ask him.

CancerFutures: The St Gallen Conferences are unique in that each time they end up delivering a new consensus about the best treatment options currently available, and these effectively become the guide-lines used for the next two years in hospitals and clinics around the world.
How did it all start?

Hans-Jörg Senn: The St Gallen Breast Cancer meetings started with our work in breast cancer. Back in 1972, I had just taken up my position here in the Kantonsspital St Gallen, and we wanted to start a programme of adjuvant treatment of breast cancer. We were on the very brink of the era of using drugs to improve cure rates in breast cancer, just about a year after Gianni Bonadonna in Milan and Bernie Fisher in the States started their programmes. At that time adjuvant treatment wasn't seen as innovative, it was seen as absolutely crazy, and we were heavily criticised by the medical oncologist community. We were ostracised for

If one centre claims to offer better treatment, you can end up with a kind of "patient tourism."

putting healthy women on chemotherapy.

Those of us who were involved in these first adjuvant breast cancer therapy trials felt that we needed to get together to exchange data and discuss results. So in 1978, we called a gathering of trialists. There were 78 of us, and that was actually the first of the St Gallen conferences.

After a few years, we decided to repeat this conference to monitor the progress of our clinical trials. So the next conference was held in 1984, and then in 1988 and so on. The consensus process was introduced at the third meeting. The conference chairpersons, Aron Goldhirsch and Richard Gelber and myself and a few others, wanted to unite all these differing results and views. And despite the objections of medical oncologists at that time, these conferences have grown ever since. To be frank, that is not what we had intended. All we wanted at the beginning was a gathering of trialists. But we began to realise that breast cancer is not just treated by trialists, but by virtually every hospital across the world.

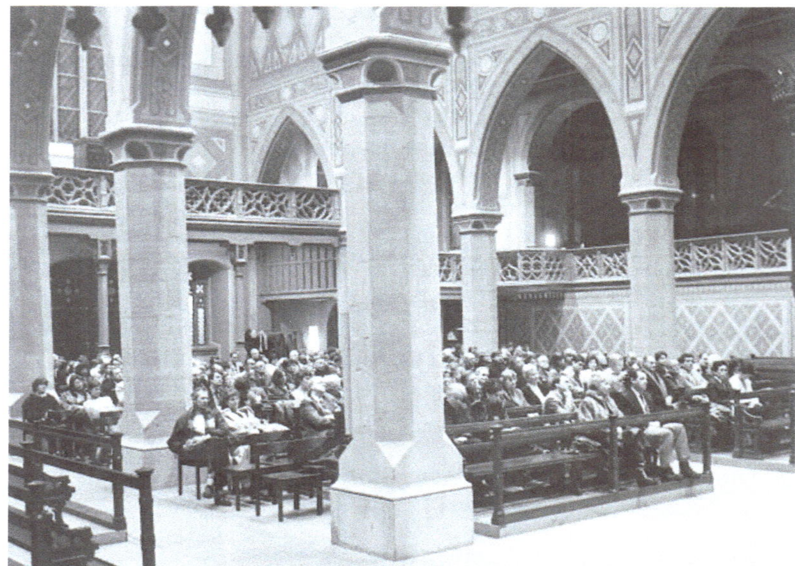

The 1990 Consensus Conference opened on a harmonious note, with a concert in the spectacular St Laurenzen Cathedral

CF: Medical oncology is a constantly changing field, with many leading authorities, and there will always be disagreement among them. Why do you think it is important to reach a consensus on the best treatment?

H-JS: The importance of consensus is that patients all over the world, or at least all over the Western world, where we have comparable medical systems, get the best treatment as recommended by international specialists on the basis of all the scientific facts available to us. If one centre claims to offer better treatment, you can end up with a kind of "patient tourism," which we don't like. The patient should get the same optimum treatment in all parts of these "comparable" systems.

CF: The requirement to reach a consensus means that the International St Gallen Guidelines necessarily err on the side of the conservative, making them perhaps slow to take on new treatments. Do you see this as a drawback?

H-JS: This is a reproach that is sometimes levelled at us. I think we are prudent. We only give out guidelines that are based on real evidence. Otherwise you risk having to retract then two years later. Two years ago we were heavily criticised for failing to reach a consensus over integrating high-dose adjuvant chemotherapy into our guidelines for treating patients at very high risk of relapse. But then one year later the South African study that had come up with strongly positive data was dis-

covered to be a scientific fraud and could not be replicated. So sometimes people who always like to be more modern can become victims of their own hopes and illusions.

That's the reason why the International St Gallen Guidelines should be evidence-based and conservative. It is up to the national health boards, oncological societies and so on to change these guidelines, or to supplement them, if they want to.

CF: Others have tried to emulate the consensus approach, in the fields of, for instance, ovarian cancer, adjuvant treatment of myeloma and melanoma, but without the same success. Can you explain how it's done?

H-JS: A team that tries to do it has to have international credibility. If we had tried this on our own, I don't think we would have been successful. In our case, the link with the

The International St Gallen Guidelines should be evidence-based and conservative.

International Breast Cancer Study Group (IBCSG) was very important. Leading members, like Aron Goldhirsch from Lugano/Milan, heavily influenced the scientific content of these conferences, and he was usually one of the chairmen of our consensus meetings held at the end. The composition of the consensus panel is also utterly important – who is in and who is out. If you do not assemble the great majority of the opinion leaders, you run the risk that those you leave out will form an "anti-consensus."

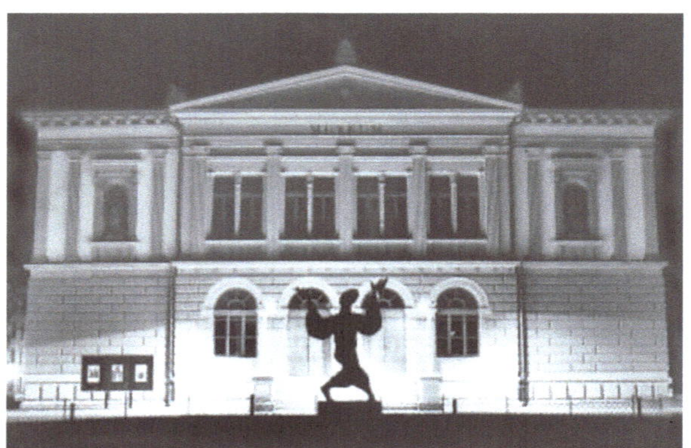

Delegates to the 1988 Consensus Conference had a chance to get to know each other at a reception in this impressive setting of the St Gallen Museum of Arts

But of course it's always a battle. When you have all these valued exponents of different ways of thinking in one panel, people like Bernard Fisher and Michael Baum, for instance, who holds some very controversial views on the issue of screening [see Masterpiece, Cancer-Futures vol 2 (7/8)], and you have three hours to get them all to come up with a set of guidelines they can all put their name to, it's not an easy task. Every time we have this battle at the end, and even after the end of the conference. But so far there has always been a result. We have managed to get the people to come to an agreement.

We also make an effort to create the right sort of atmosphere. We encourage delegates to explore the culture of the city and the beauty of the area, and to get to know one another on a social level. We offer the speakers the chance to spend a few days skiing. So it's not only scientific exchange and battling. I think this can help. I am certainly told that there is a certain aura around this conference.

CF: Where would you like to see the St Gallen Conferences going from here?

H-JS: When the Conferences first started, 25 years ago, mastectomy was standard, at least on this continent, and adjuvant chemotherapy was something that came after surgery, stuck on like a pigtail. Now breast-conserving "lesser" surgery is standard, and adjuvant therapy has become the main part. So things change, and we have to change accordingly. For instance, the Conference has now changed its title from Adjuvant Therapy of Breast Cancer, to Primary Therapy of Breast Cancer, to reflect an increasingly multi-model view that incorporates into the consensus everything on the treatment of early breast cancer, whether it is surgical, or radiological, or chemo- or hormone therapy.

I would like to see breast cancer prevention becoming a central focus. This is a gap in medical oncology that I have become increasingly aware of during my long period working in hospitals. While we need to find the best treatment for advanced disease and supportive care, it would, of course, be far better to avoid disease, or at least to avoid extensive disease, to discover it early and to treat it with a less traumatic impact on the patient. Here in St Gallen, we are part of the first international trials of chemoprevention of breast cancer, which involves giving chemotherapy to healthy people who genetically or through family history are at very high risk of developing cancer, in order to stop the disease developing at all, or at least delay its onset. I think this will be a big thing in the future.

CF: When you see the International St Gallen Guidelines adopted as national guidelines in many European countries, and used as the handbook for treatment in hospitals from Australia to the UK, how do you feel about your personal role in it all?

H-JS: I would be lying if I were to say I am not proud of it. It is a practical contribution that we in St Gallen have been able to offer the oncology world.

CF: Another very practical contribution of yours has been to champion the cause of the patient's quality of life. You organised the first international conference on supportive care and launched the journal Supportive Care in Oncology. What made you take up this issue?

H-JS: To be honest it was our nurses, particularly our head nurse Dr Agnes Glaus, who persuaded me to do something about it.

It was around the mid-1980s. I'd had the great privilege of living through the age of discovery of many new cytostatic drugs that could cure disseminated cancers such as leukaemia and lymphoma, as well as testicular cancer metastasising to the lungs, and so on. Many people were convinced that this process would go on, and we would find ways to cure everything that disseminates. But around this time, many of us began to realise that this process was beginning to plateau out, and that we had a lot of patients for whom treatment would remain palliative.

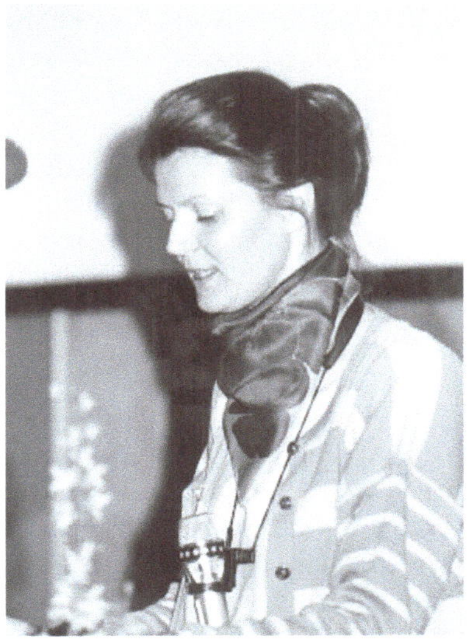

Dr Agnes Glaus, head nurse at the St Gallen Tumour Centre, was one of the first to argue the case for supportive care

We could, perhaps, keep them in remission, but there were side-effects. And so the balance between effects

I would like to see breast cancer prevention becoming a central focus.

and side effects was coming increasingly into question.

CF: So what did you do?

H-JS: In February 1987 we assembled all the people we could find in the literature who treated and managed pain, or nausea and vomiting, or infections – all the aspects of supportive care which make the patient's life more agreeable – and we called the first meeting of Supportive Care in Cancer Patients. There were more than 700 people, about half of them nurses – specialist nurses, academically trained nurses, from America, Australia, about 75 countries in all. And that was the start of "supportive care" at the international level.

In a way we were victims of our own success, because within one year there were two more first international meetings on supportive care in cancer, which were virtual copies of ours. One of these was called by an American conference organiser, who took our name and branded it for themselves. That's why we ended up calling ourselves the Multinational Association of Supportive Care in Cancer (MASCC).

The big mistake we made was that we did not create a society at that initial meeting, because, apart from problems caused by people trying to copy us, we ended up losing ground to the palliative care movement, which was focusing attention almost exclusively on pain, whereas we were trying to draw attention to the need to treat the whole range of disease symptoms, such as infectious complications, anaemia and nausea and vomiting. Happily, over the years, many of the differences between the palliative care movement, with its emphasis on taking incurable patients out of treatment, and our vision of supportive care within a treatment setting, have lessened.

CF: What progress has been made in supportive care since that first meeting?

H-JS: From the initial meeting we set up a journal, Supportive Care in Cancer, dedicated to exploring the new field of supportive care and stimulating thinking about how we can benefit patients. I think we managed to get the issue onto the agenda, because today supportive care is no longer only talked about by us, but it is discussed at the major medical oncology conferences.

Important progress has also been made in new treatments. The Italian Society of Medical Oncology, for instance, has done great work on anti-emetics. Another important development is the injection of growth factors to stimulate erythropoiesis or leukopoiesis in the bone marrow, curing anaemia, or leukopaenia, or infection. And this of course means that industry is starting to take more of an interest, and is bringing more funding into this aspect of cancer care, because supportive care now represents a market for them. Previously, lack of funding was a real problem, and we struggled initially to find enough backing to launch the journal.

CF: At what level do you see pressure for change being most effective? Would European Guidelines on supportive care encourage change in health systems that have been slower to take supportive care on board?

H-JS: The change needs to come from a national level, because, unlike breast cancer, which poses a more technical problem, supportive care has a lot of psychosocial and emotional involvement and social and cultural differences play a much bigger role. For instance, "truth telling" is different in southern Europe than in northern Europe. As the editor of Supportive Care in Cancer, every third month or so I get a paper from Turkey or Greece or from another southern country that tells us that 79% or 85% of the population would not like to be told if they had a bad prognosis. This is completely contrary to what is going on here and in the US. We don't understand each other on this level. We cannot copy each other's systems.

There are also legal differences. Pain treatment, for example, will vary because there are still countries even in Europe where all opiates remain illegal. Euthanasia is another issue that differs in both the cultural and the legal approach from country to country. So I think European Guidelines could be effective, but only if they are drawn up by panels in which all the countries are truly represented, which is often not the case.

CF: Where would you like to see the supportive care movement going?

H-JS: We would like to see more medical oncologists and oncology nurses taking up the issues, and to see supportive care featuring more prominently in their meetings. I think there remains a certain passive resistance – perhaps because it is still confused with the early palliative care movement, so some people feel there is a contradiction between supportive care and the primary task of curing patients, which there is not. It's all part of the same holistic approach. Unfortunately, the system changes slowly. I would like to see much faster progress in getting medical oncologists to embrace the concept of supportive care.

CF: Finally, I'd like to address the question of language and communication. You were instrumental in setting up the first German-language courses for the European School of Oncology (ESO) – the Deutsch-

sprachiges Programm. What prompted this?

H-JS: When I'm teaching, I've found that English is all very well when you are dealing with purely scientific, medical subjects, but you run into problems when you want to discuss personal, emotional, or spiritual issues. This can only be done in

I would like to see much faster progress in getting medical oncologists to embrace the concept of supportive care.

your mother tongue. Also English is little use when teaching oncology nurses, because, at least in continental Europe, nurses are vocationally trained, and their En-glish is often not good enough. It was an ESO conference in Vienna that finally convinced me of the need to run some courses in German. Almost all of the 75 nurses and physicians attending were German speakers, and yet there we were, trying to conduct a discussion in English. It was not only impossible, it was ridiculous.

So about seven years ago we started introducing the more practical courses – on social aspects of care, palliative care, supportive care

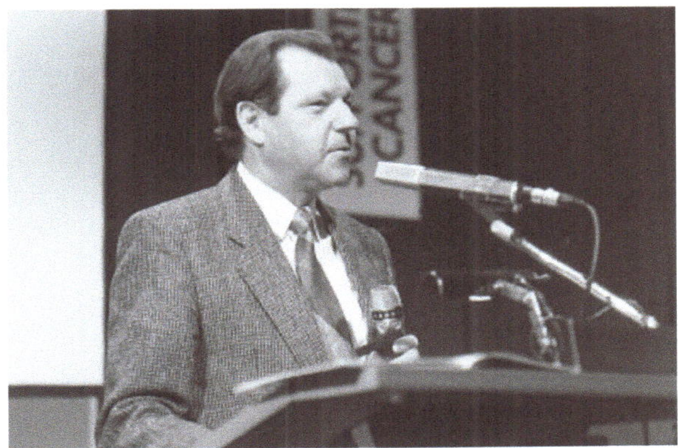

and nursing courses – in German. We were not the first – there were already ESO courses running in French and Spanish – but we are now the most flourishing language section of ESO. We run 15 or 16 courses every year, and they are very popular.

CF: Language continues to be a barrier to working at a pan-European level, and the picture is becoming more complicated as more countries join the European Union. Do you think more language programmes could be a solution for other language groups?

H-JS: Not necessarily. First of all, programmes have to be efficient and economically viable, because they take time and money to organise. It works in German, because there are more than 100 million people in Europe who speak this language – more than French and Spanish put together. But you couldn't do the same, for instance, for Bulgarian or Romanian. The issue of quality is also crucial. ESO courses are based on the most up-to-date evidence-based knowledge, and all teaching staff are highly regarded within medical oncology. We don't want that to be jeopardised by further language diversification. The English language courses will always remain at the core of the ESO curriculum; while the other language programmes are important, they can play only a supplementary role.

Gianni Bonnadona: Fighting for Every Life

ANNA WAGSTAFF

With 33 major awards to his name, Professor Gianni Bonadonna, Director of the Division of Oncology of the Istituto Nazionale Tumori in Milan until 1998, and now chair of their Prospective Clinical Trials Committee, must be the single most decorated hero of medical oncology. He carried out the first trials of adriamycin, "the most important cancer medicine of our generation," and he developed the ABVD (adriamycin, bleomycin, vinblastine and dacarbazine) combination, which remains the gold standard for treating Hodgkin's disease. His patients were the first ever to receive adjuvant treatment with CMF (cyclophosphamide, methotrexate, fluorouracil), and almost 30 years on many of the first trial cohort of 386 remain in regular contact, providing the longest data curves in the business. He was at the forefront of the battle to convince the surgical establishment which then ruled supreme in the cancer world that adjuvant therapy could make a real difference. He is now the first to conduct trials using various sequential regimens. He is a scientist's scientist. But he is also a patient's doctor. And when Anna Wagstaff went to hear the story of his amazing career, he had this message for the younger generation: "Don't get too caught up in the deluge of data and statistics: it's time to reconnect with the patient."

CancerFutures: CMF is the regimen that first convinced a sceptical oncology world of the benefits of adjuvant treatment, and it emains to this day the gold standard against which other regimens are compared. How did it all begin?

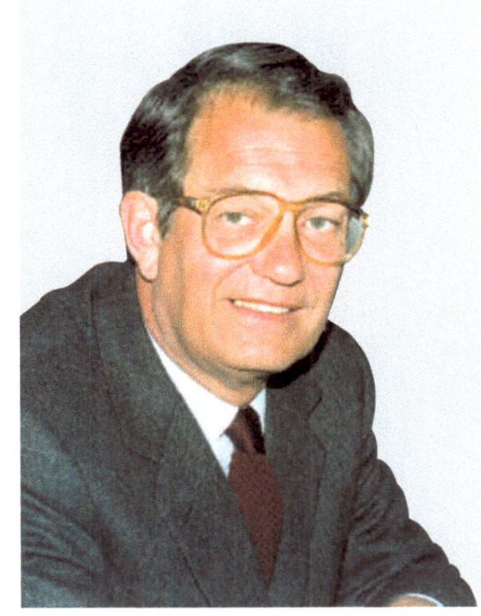

Gianni Bonnadona: The story of CMF started in 1972. I was at that time Associate Director of the Division of Clinical Oncology here at the Istituto Nazionale Tumori, and was invited to visit the US National Cancer Institute (NCI) by Paul Carbone. Things were beginning to move in medical oncology in the US, and among all the reports that I saw on that visit were three separate studies that formed the basis for the work I was later to undertake. I read the early results of a quadruple drug regimen, cyclophosphamide, methotrexate, fluorouracil and prednisone (CMFP), that was showing a remarkable response rate in clinically disseminated breast cancer. I also read the study protocol of the Eastern Cooperative Oncology Group, which was randomly testing

I was convinced adjuvant therapy was worth a try.

CMF versus melphalan (PAM) in advanced breast cancer. The third piece of the jigsaw was an early draft of the National Surgical Adjuvant Breast Project (NSABP) trial, led by Bernie Fisher, on radical mastectomy versus radical mastectomy followed by adjuvant PAM in node-positive breast cancer.

I was convinced adjuvant therapy was worth a try, and I discussed with Paul Carbone the possibility of conducting trials with CMF in Milan. I got the backing of the Milan Institute and of the NCI, which provided much of the funding – the first funding ever for a trial conducted outside the US. By June 1973 CMF had proved its worth in advanced disease both in efficacy and lower toxicity compared with other regimens, and we were ready to start the adjuvant trials. Over the next two years 386 patients were enrolled in the study.

CF: Was there a lot of excitement over what these first trials might come up with?

GB: No. At that time nobody was interested. Cancer treatment in those days was entirely about surgery, and the surgeons, with the exception of Professor Veronesi, the chief surgeon here in Milan, and of course Bernie Fisher who was leading the US trials, were not just scep-

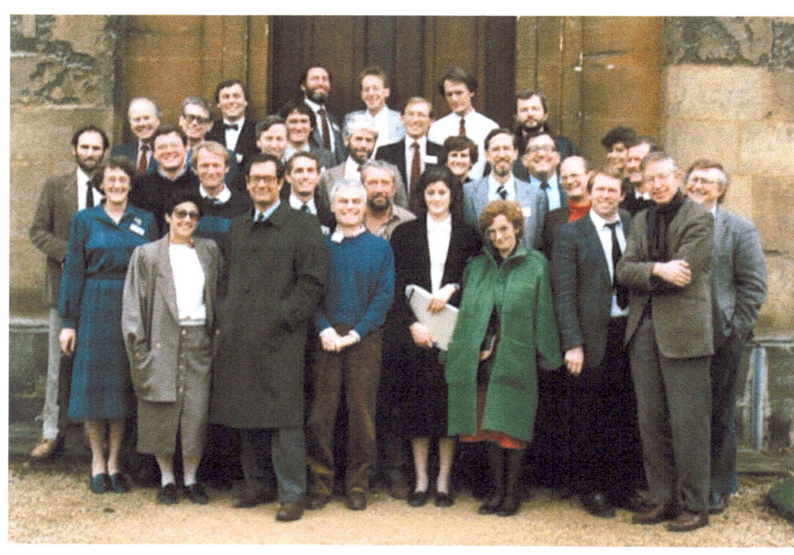

tical, they were hostile. We were left completely alone.

For us, the logic was clear: we knew from previous data that chemotherapy was more effective the earlier you caught the disease. So we reasoned that if we could catch metastatic lesions at such an early stage that they were not yet detectable, the cure rate could be even higher. But the surgeons didn't want to know. At the time there were very few chemotherapists, and they were not rated highly; the attitude among surgeons was: "Chemotherapists deliver drugs in advanced disease and try to define whether there is complete disappearance of the tumour or a reduction of the lesion. Surgeons operate and we have complete remission for the entire life of the patient."

Of course we knew that this was not true, but in those days surgeons were really not aware of how many of their patients relapsed and, in particular, how many went on to develop metastases, because the majority of their patients were never followed up. Even patients who later returned to the Institute for further treatment would come to us in the chemotherapy department or perhaps be sent for radiotherapy. The surgeons rarely saw their patients again, and I think they didn't want to hear about how many patients were being failed by surgery alone. It was a matter of prestige.

CF: And after the preliminary results were published?

GB: The early results were very positive. Before adjuvant therapy, less than 50% of patients with node-positive breast cancer remained disease free at three years. We managed

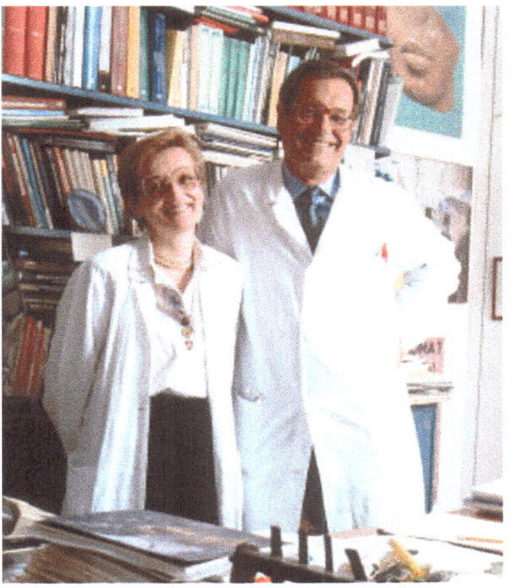

With Pinuccia Valagussa, Head of Operations for Clinical Trials, who has worked with Bonnadona for almost 30 years. They have been through many trials together

to increase that to 62%. We presented the results at a meeting of the European Organisation for Research and Treatment of Cancer (EORTC) in Brussels in 1975 – the first EORTC meeting on breast cancer. Even then there was great scepticism. But on the flight home, it became clear that the results really had begun to spark some excitement, and many who had remained silent at the meeting started to pump us for more information.

Among the most resistant to taking on board our evidence at that time were the British. But soon after our results were published in the New England Medical Journal in September of the following year, John Hayward and Bob Rubens from the Royal Marsden in London visited us and asked if they could conduct an audit of all the data from our trial. They were convinced by what they saw, and the support of John Hayward, in particular, an internationally respected surgeon, proved a real turning point. After that there were fewer objections.

Another important milestone was the International Overview conducted by a group in Oxford starting in 1982–83. One problem with proving the efficacy of a treatment was simply getting enough data to prove statistical significance. The Oxford Early Breast Cancer Trialists' Collaborative Group were the first to try to collate and then analyse the figures from all the trials into adjuvant treatment – both chemo and hormonal – across the world. The results provided the most convincing evidence for the benefits of adjuvant therapy. The first complete analysis was run in 1985 and published in 1988.

CF: Did you expect CMF still to be in use 30 years on, and do you agree with those who argue that the much more aggressive therapies which have subsequently come into use end up overtreating too many women when used in an adjuvant setting?

GB: All the effort has to be to improve the cure rate. We now know for certain that there are more effective treatments than CMF, for instance administering four cycles of adriamycin followed by CMF, which is one of the sequential treatments we have been trialling here in Milan. In my view we must recommend

All the effort has to be improve the curerate.

whatever is most effective, despite the somewhat higher levels of toxicity. I know there are still some people who favour CMF, but I think it should be reserved for patients who cannot safely take the more toxic drugs, for instance if they have a concomitant heart condition.

You have to remember that when we started with CMF, there were no supportive treatments available. Nowadays, although certain doses of adriamycin and the taxanes do carry a high risk of causing neutropaenia, for instance, we can deliver growth factors to counter this risk. We are also able to deliver anti-emetics to combat the higher levels of nausea and vomiting induced by these more toxic drugs. The main thing is that we explain to patients about the relative effectiveness and the side-effects of alternative treatments and give them the option.

Of course, in any adjuvant chemotherapy programme there will always be some patients who undergo treatment who would never have relapsed anyway, and who therefore end up being "overtreated". But the point is that, beyond some basic prognostic factors, we still have no reliable way of telling them apart from those who will benefit from the treatment.

Even here progress is being made. For instance, there is a lot of interest now in HER2 receptor over-expression as an indication that the tumour is sensitive to treatment with adriamycin and taxanes. However, it is also clear that adriamycin has an effect even where there is no over-expression of the HER2 receptor, so at the moment at least we cannot rule out adriamycin for these patients.

Clearly advances in genetic profiling will also be very important in helping us tailor the treatment to the tumour, and this is the way to address the problem of overtreatment.

CF: Adriamycin, of course, also began its clinical life here at the

Milan Institute, and went on to form a part of the ABVD regime developed by you, which remains the gold standard for treating Hodgkin's disease.

GB: Adriamycin was a milestone. It was the first drug to show that it is possible to cure some advanced cancers. It was developed by Farmitalia, an Italian drug company, and we conducted the first trials in patients with advanced inoperable sarcoma here at the Institute. The results were pretty dramatic.

I remember the first patient ever to receive the drug. He was a young man with a very large advanced sarcoma, and had been enrolled in the phase I clinical trial at the Institute. He came into my study three days after the medicine had been delivered, and he was completely bald. This was pretty shocking at the time. We knew, and we always advised patients, that chemotherapy drugs result in hair loss, but never before had we seen it on this scale. The effect was so traumatic that he decided to discontinue the treatment. But luckily we found that in those same three days the effect on the tumour had been equally dramatic – it was reducing at a remarkable rate. So he agreed to continue the treatment. I felt that this was a real breakthrough. For the first time we had a drug that actually managed to cure some patients with advanced cancer.

When the Director of the Institute first caught sight of the patients on my ward as he was doing his rounds, he turned to me with a quizzical look and said: "Dott. Bonadonna, tutti calvi nel suo reparto? [Doctor Bonadonna, all bald on your ward?]" He then asked, "Do you feel

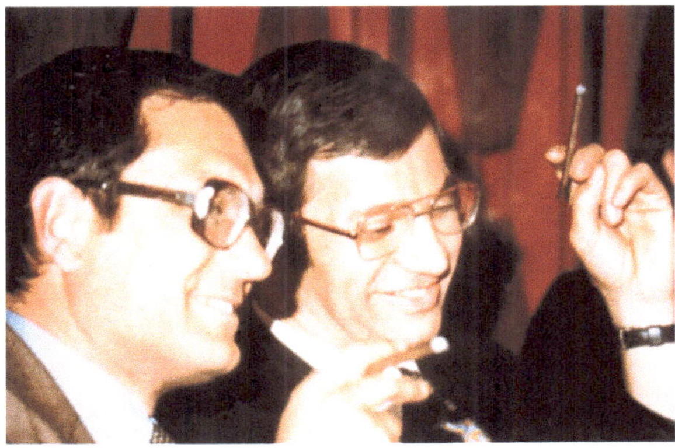

With Vince De Vita (right), who developed the MOPP regimen for Hodgkin's disease. Bonadonna sees his own development of the ABDV regimen, which improved the cure rate in Hodgkin's from around 60% to 80–85%, as his greatest achievement

this new drug is going to cure patients? Well go ahead!"

I believe it is the most important cancer medicine of our generation, because it was the first that delivered a high cure rate in many types of cancer, with moderate toxicity. Not only did it prove effective in advanced sarcoma that had previously been incurable, but it was also very active in malignant lymphomas, in advanced breast cancer and in paediatric tumours. When the first patient was treated, in September 1968, there were other drugs available, but none that could compare with the level of shrinkage of the neoplastic lesion achieved by adriamycin.

It was a few years after that first trial that I developed the ABVD (adriamycin, bleomycin, vinblastine and dacarbazine) combination for Hodgkin's disease, which has a cure rate of between 80 and 85%. This was a huge improvement on the cure rate offered by the then gold standard MOPP (mechloretamine, vincristine, procarbazine, prednisone) regimen, which had been developed by my friend and colleague Vincent de Vita in the US, and at that time had a 60% cure rate. I consider it my greatest achievement.

CF: Your work has earned you 33 major oncology awards, making you one of the world's most celebrated medical oncologists. What advice do you have for the next generation?

GB: The message I want to pass on above all others is to remember

I worry about the "scientification" of medical oncology.

that you are treating a human being and not just a disease. I know that the medical oncology training of today stresses the need to interact with the patient much more than perhaps it used to do when I was a trainee, but there are many pressures working in the opposite direction.

I worry about the "scientification" of medical oncology. The proliferation of studies and data has of course led to hugely important advances in treatment; we know

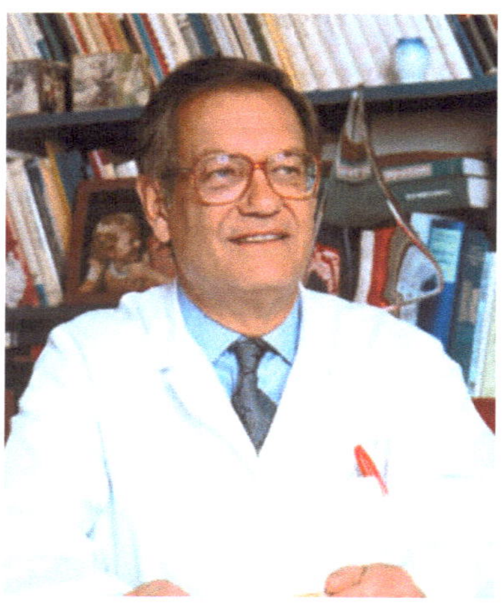

more about the disease and more about treatments. But there is a danger that physicians take all the data curves and significance values as their starting point and simply try to fit each patient into the correct slot, rather than understanding that cancer is something the doctor and the patient need to fight together. Medicine is an art not a science.

It's not just a question of personal attitudes, it's the number of obstacles that get in the way of the doctor–patient relationship. Nowadays it's a big job simply keeping up with developments in the field and, within the new multidisciplinary approach, today's medical oncologist is expected to be familiar and communicate with not only surgeons, radiotherapists, pathologists and radiologists, but increasingly with biologists, geneticists, and even information scientists and statisticians. How much time does that leave to communicate with patients?

The pressure to publish can also distort priorities at the expense of patients, which wouldn't be so bad if every paper represented a real step forward in our scientific understanding, but this is increasingly not so.

It was once the case that we would publish only if we had something to say, either positive or negative, that had real implications either for the patient, for the profession or for society. But nowadays people are writing papers just for the sake of being published, and, as a reviewer for many journals in the field, I find more and more papers that don't seem to have any point to them. They have some data, they pass it through the SPSS or SAS statistical software package, and they submit it for publication. The median follow-up period of randomised studies of adjuvant chemotherapy published today is only three years, and many of these studies are never heard of again. What can you say about an adjuvant drug after only three years? Breast cancer is a chronic disease, and we are still gathering data on the CMF trials 30 years on.

The problem is that today's medical oncologists are having to make their way in a system in which the number of papers you publish, and the "impact factor" this gives you, is the key to getting the job you want and the funding for your research. Publish or perish.

With all these other pressures, we find that here in Milan, doctors have only about five hours in which to see around 20, or even 22 ambulatory patients, and even then much of the consultation is spent dealing with endless bureaucracy. As a result patients are too often simply being handed written information when asked to give their consent to treatment, without anyone taking the time to sit down and discuss it with them. So even if the training today is all about being more patient-centred, the reality is that the patient is being increasingly squeezed out. This is dreadful and really has to change.

CF: Eight years ago, you suffered a cerebral haemorrhage so serious that everyone assumed your career was over. What happened?

GB: In October 1995 it was like the atom bomb exploded in my hands. From the perspective of any scientifically derived probability curve, the damage I sustained left me little hope of returning to work. However, having spent my life fighting alongside patients who were themselves battling against desperation, misery, fear and despair, I was determined to find the strength to fight for myself. And with the help and support of those around me, I got myself back into working order and returned to doing the job I love. I hope that my experience can offer encouragement to everyone who has experienced or who is still battling with a traumatic disease.

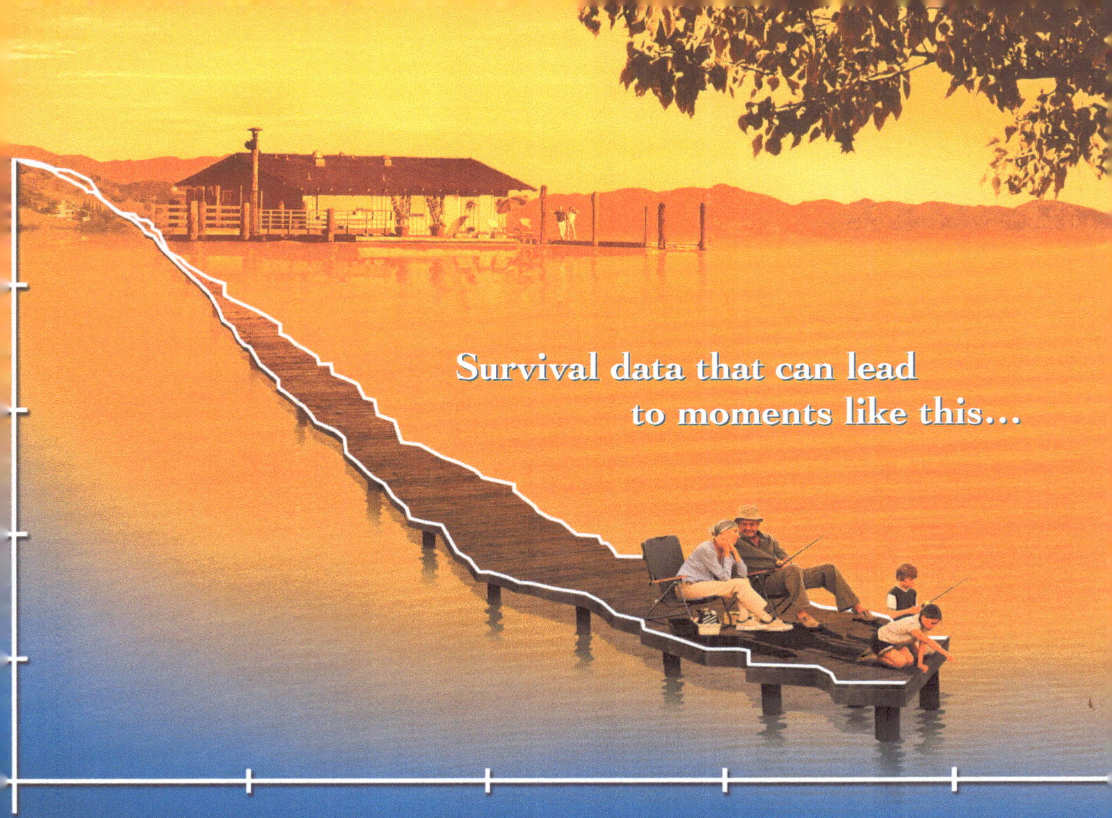

- Overall survival advantage in metastatic breast cancer and as first-line therapy in advanced non-small cell lung cancer[1-5]

- A manageable safety profile[6]

- Improved quality of life demonstrated in patients with lung cancer[4,5]*

- Most convenient taxane available — 1-hour IV infusion[6]

Please see brief summary of full prescribing information on the adjacent page.

*In breast cancer studies, Taxotere® demonstrated quality of life comparable to comparators.[1,3]

References: 1. Nabholtz J-M, Senn HJ, Bezwoda WR, et al. Prospective randomized trial of docetaxel versus mitomycin plus vinblastine in patients with metastatic breast cancer progressing despite previous anthracycline-containing chemotherapy. *J Clin Oncol.* 1999;17:1413-1424. **2.** Ravdin P, Erban J, Overmoyer B, et al. Phase III comparison of docetaxel (D) and paclitaxel (P) in patients with metastatic breast cancer (MBC). Presented at: 12th Annual European Cancer Conference; September 21–25, 2003; Copenhagen, Denmark. Abstract 670. **3.** Jones S, Erban J, Overmoyer B, et al, and the TAX 311 Clinical Trialists. Phase III comparison of docetaxel and paclitaxel in patients with metastatic breast cancer. Slide presentation at: 26th Annual San Antonio Breast Cancer Symposium; December 3–6, 2003; San Antonio, Tex. **4.** Fossella F, Pereira JR, von Pawel J, et al. Randomized, multinational, phase III study of docetaxel plus platinum combinations versus vinorelbine plus cisplatin for advanced non–small-cell lung cancer: the TAX 326 Study Group. *J Clin Oncol.* 2003;21:3016-3024. **5.** Kubota K, Watanabe K, Kunitoh H, et al. Phase III randomized trial of docetaxel plus cisplatin versus vindesine plus cisplatin in patients with stage IV non–small-cell lung cancer: the Japanese Taxotere Lung Cancer Study Group. *J Clin Oncol.* 2004;22:254-261. **6.** Taxotere® Abbreviated Prescribing Information. Antony, France: Aventis Pharma S.A.; February 2004.

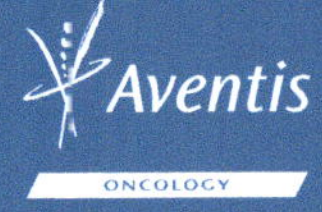

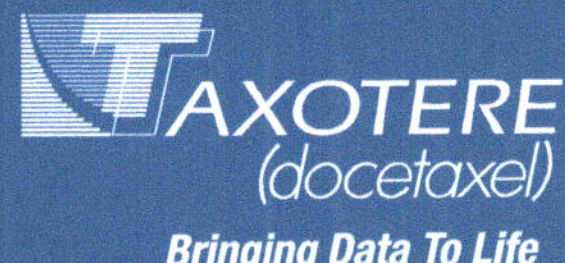

©2004 Aventis Pharmaceuticals Inc.

10/04

TAXOTERE®
(docetaxel)

ABBREVIATED PRESCRIBING INFORMATION for TAXOTERE® (docetaxel) 20 or 80 mg

TAXOTERE® (docetaxel) concentrate for solution for infusion is available in single-dose vials containing 20 or 80 mg in 0.5 or 2.0 ml of polysorbate 80, respectively with a solvent vial (13% ethanol in water for injections).

PHARMACOLOGICAL PROPERTIES:

Docetaxel promotes the assembly of tubulin into stable microtubules and inhibits their disassembly.

INDICATIONS:

Locally advanced or metastatic breast cancer in combination with doxorubicin in patients who have not previously received cytotoxic therapy, or in combination with capecitabine after failure of cytotoxic therapy, which should have included an anthracycline. Locally advanced or metastatic breast as monotherapy after failure of cytotoxic therapy, which should have included an anthracycline or alkylating agent. Locally advanced or metastatic non-small cell lung cancer (NSCLC) in combination with cisplatin for patients who have not received prior cytotoxic therapy for this condition, or as monotherapy after failure of prior chemotherapy.

DOSAGE:

75 mg/m² in combination therapy with doxorubicin (50 mg/m²) for breast cancer. 100 mg/m² for breast cancer and 75 mg/m² for NSCLC, as a one-hour infusion every three weeks. All patients must be pretreated with an oral corticosteroid for 3 days starting one day before each TAXOTERE administration. **Dosage adjustments during treatment:** TAXOTERE should be administered when the neutrophil count is ≥ 1,500 cells/mm³. In patients with either febrile neutropenia, neutrophil < 500 cells/mm³ for > 7 days, severe or cumulative cutaneous reactions or severe neurosensory signs and/or symptoms, the dose should be reduced by 25%. If these reactions continue, the dosage should either be decreased to 60 mg or treatment discontinued. No data are available in patients with hepatic impairment treated by docetaxel in combination. **Dosage adjustments in patients with elevated liver function tests:** Patients with elevated ALT and/or AST > 1.5 times the upper limit of the normal range (ULN) concurrent with increases in alkaline phosphatase > 2.5 times the ULN, the recommended dose of TAXOTERE is 75 mg/m². In patients with serum bilirubin > ULN and/or ALT/AST values > 3.5 times the ULN associated with alkaline phosphatase > 6 times the ULN, TAXOTERE should not be used unless strictly indicated.

CONTRAINDICATIONS:

Hypersensitivity reactions to docetaxel or polysorbate 80; Baseline neutrophil count of < 1,500 cells/mm³; Severe liver impairment; Pregnancy or breast feeding.

WARNINGS AND PRECAUTIONS: Haematology: Neutropenia is the most frequent adverse reaction and may require dosage reduction (see Dosage adjustments). Frequent monitoring of complete blood counts is required in all patients receiving docetaxel. **Severe hypersensitivity** reactions require immediate discontinuation and appropriate therapy and should not be rechallenged. Minor **hypersensitivity** reactions do not require interruption of therapy. **Cutaneous and CNS:** Localised skin erythema or severe neurosensory signs and/or symptoms may lead to dosage reduction, or treatment interruption or discontinuation. **Fluid retention:** Corticosteroid premedication can reduce the incidence and severity of fluid retention. Patients with pleural effusion, pericardial effusion and ascites should be monitored closely. **Liver function tests** (LFTs) should be measured at baseline and before each cycle. **Contraceptive** measures must be taken during and for > 3 months after therapy.

INTERACTIONS:

Caution when treating patients with drugs metabolized by cytochrome P450-3A.

SIDE EFFECTS:

(In patients at 100 mg/m² single agent and 75 mg/m² in combination, respectively): **Haematology:** Severe neutropenia (76.4% and 91.7%); Fever with severe neutropenia (11.8% and 34.1%); Infectious episodes (20% with 5.7% severe, and 35.3% with 7.8% severe); Thrombocytopenia (7.8% and 28.1%); Anemia (90.4% with 8.9% severe and 96.1% with 9.4% severe). **Hypersensitivity** reactions (25.9% with 5.3% severe and 4.7% with 1.2% severe) resolved after discontinuing the infusion and appropriate therapy. Reversible **cutaneous** reactions (56.6% and 13.6%) with 73% of these events reversed within 21 days; Nail disorders (27.9% and 20.2%). **Fluid retention** (64.1% with 6.5% severe and 35.7% with 1.2% severe). The median cumulative dose to onset was 818.9 mg/m². The median cumulative dose to treatment discontinuation was more than 1.000 mg/m². **Gastrointestinal:** Nausea (40.5% and 64%); Vomiting (24.5% and 45%); Diarrhea (40.6% and 45.7%); Anorexia (16.8% and 8.5%); Constipation (9.8% and 14.3%);

Stomatitis (41.8% and 58.1%); **Neuro-sensory** signs and/or symptoms (50% with 4.1% severe and 30.2% with 0.4% severe) and **neuro-motor** events (13.8% with 4% severe and 2.3% with 0.4% severe). The events were spontaneously reversible within 3 months in 35.3% Pts. **Cardiovascular:** Hypotension (3.8% and 0.4%); Dysrhythmia (4.1% and 1.2%). **Infusion site reactions** were generally mild and occurred in 5.6% and 3.1% Pts, respectively. **LFTs** Increases in AST, ALT, bilirubin and alkaline phosphatase > 2.5 times the ULN were observed in < 5% Pts treated at 100 mg/m². In patients treated in combination, less than 1% of patients experienced grade 3-4 increase in AST, ALT and grade 3-4 increase in bilirubin and alkaline phosphatase were observed in less than 2.5% of the patients. **Others:** Alopecia (79% and 94.6%); Severe asthenia (11.2% and 8.1%); Myalgias (20% and 8.5%); Pain (16.5% and 17.1%). **Continuing Surveillance:** Rare cases of dehydration as a consequence of gastrointestinal events, gastrointestinal perforation, neutropenic enterocolitis, venous thromboembolic events, myocardial infarction, pulmonary oedema in association with fluid retention, acute respiratory distress syndrome, interstitial pneumonia and radiation recall phenomenon.

CLINICAL:

Two randomized phase III comparative studies, involving respectively 326 alkylating and 392 anthracycline failure metastatic breast cancer Pts, have been performed with docetaxel at the dose of 100 mg/m² every 3 weeks. In anthracycline failure Pts, the response rate (RR) was 33% with TAXOTERE versus 12% with a combination of mitomycin and vinblastine. TAXOTERE prolonged the time to progression (TPP) (19 weeks versus 11 weeks) and the overall survival (11 months versus 9 months). In alkylating failure Pts, the RR was 52% with TAXOTERE versus 37% with doxorubicin. The TPP was prolonged (27 weeks with TAXOTERE versus 23 weeks with doxorubicin), and the time to response was shortened (12 weeks versus 23 weeks). One large randomized phase III study (429 previously untreated metastatic breast cancer Pts) has been performed with doxorubicin (50 mg/m²) in combination with docetaxel (75 mg/m²) versus doxorubicin (60 mg/m²) in combination with cyclophosphamide (600 mg/m²): median TPP (37.3 weeks versus 31.9 weeks), overall RR (59.3% versus 46.5%). In one phase III study, in previously treated NSCLC patients, time to progression (12.3 weeks versus 7 weeks) and overall survival were significantly longer for docetaxel at 75 mg/m² compared to Best Supportive Care (BSC). The 1-year survival rate was also significantly longer in docetaxel (40%) versus BSC (16%). There was less use of morphinic analgesic (p<0.001), non-morphinic analgesics (p<0.01), other disease-related medications (p=0.06) and radiotherapy (p<0.01) in patients treated with docetaxel at 75 mg/m² compared to those with BSC. The overall response rate was 6.8% in the evaluable patients, and the median duration of response was 26.1 weeks. **KINETICS** are dose-independent. Excretion is mainly faecal following hepatic metabolism. Docetaxel is > 95% protein bound. In a population pharmacokinetic analysis neither age nor sex had an impact on kinetics; there was a 27% decrease in total clearance in patients with elevated LFTs.

PRECLINICAL:

Docetaxel is mutagenic consistent with its pharmacological activity. **SHELF-LIFE:** Vials should be stored between +2°C and +25°C and protected from bright light. The shelf-life is respectively 18 and 24 months for TAXOTERE 20 and 80 mg.

INSTRUCTIONS FOR USE:

TAXOTERE must be diluted with the entire contents of the solvent vial. TAXOTERE premix solution (10 mg docetaxel/ml) unless used immediately to prepare the infusion solution, can be stored for up to 8 hours either between +2°C and +8°C or at room temperature. To prepare, inject the appropriate amount of TAXOTERE premix solution into a 250 ml infusion bag or bottle containing either 0.9% sodium chloride solution or 5% glucose solution to produce a final concentration not exceeding 0.74 mg/ml. Use the infusion solution within the 4 hours.

MARKETING AUTHORISATION HOLDER:

Aventis Pharma S.A. 20 avenue Raymond Aron 92165 Antony Cedex France **AUTHORISATION NUMBERS:** EU/1/95/002/001 and EU/1/95/002/002 **DATE OF FIRST AUTHORISATION:** November 1995.

DATE OF REVISION:

February 2004. See European Summary of Product Characteristics for further information.

©2004 Aventis Pharma S.A. Antony, France

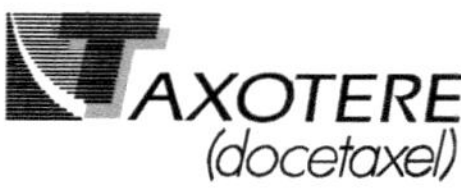

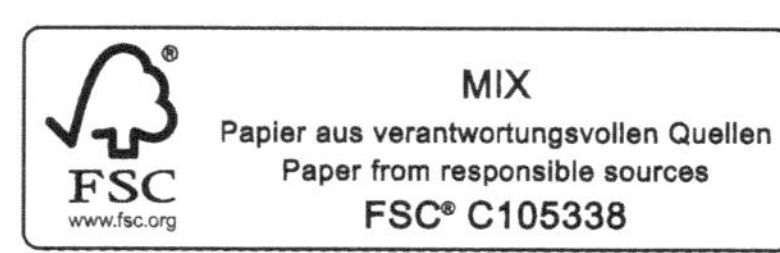

If you have any concerns about our products,
you can contact us on
ProductSafety@springernature.com

In case Publisher is established outside the EU,
the EU authorized representative is:
Springer Nature Customer Service Center GmbH
Europaplatz 3, 69115 Heidelberg, Germany

Printed by Libri Plureos GmbH
in Hamburg, Germany